Also by Dr Teddy Andrew Mulenga

The Sceptic, vol1

Brooms

Life's Pitfalls

Sleep Your Way to Success-Study Made Simple

Ripples in the Sky

About This and That

Welcome to Livingstone

Lamentations

Confessions of a doctor

The Fourth Testament

Inside out

ISBN-13: 978-1981628858

ISBN-10: 1981628851

Printed in USA.
Published at Mvibe Media Mosi-a Tunya House old wing, Room 312,
Email mvibemedia@yahoo.com
Livingstone

Dedication

To all my former patients, my friends and colleagues, I dedicate this book. To my patients you had to be sick to educate me, to my friends and colleagues, we all stood together as we treated our patients.

Acknowledgements

I should thank all my staff, at Mvibe Media, for the good hours spent perfecting my book. Special thanks go to Wilson Kalofya for having spent so many hours with me poring over the fine prints day in day out looking for that special misspelling that always escapes the writer once in a while .However, any omissions, that could have escaped notice, are duly acknowledged as squarely my own

Contents

Introduction

Health it should be said is the most valuable diamond an individual can have. You can buy a car, love, a house, food but you can't buy health. This is the reason everybody dies, the reason no one has ever come out of this life alive! Health is a condition when the human body is operating at its best, physically and mentally. Some may say it is the absence of disease. This is a condition that humans tend to value when they lose it, more than anything else. Something WHO calls a complete presence of physical and mental wellbeing. Difficult to define, but we all know when we are feeling better and when we feel like vomiting out all our insides!

  This of course is not a book for doctors and nurses to use as a text book. It's for every one of us to discuss with me health issues in a less dramatic, in a more common language, the common diseases and conditions that we find ourselves grappling with. Something tells me that you do not need to go to a medical school in order to appreciate what disease is; you don't have to go to medical school to learn how to be sick!

I must mention that the idea to write this book for all came as a result of the phone calls I used to get when I was doing a radio phone- in programme in Livingstone at Zambezi FM and Falls Fem. realized then that sometimes- common sense is not so common after all and what we the trained in medicine take for granted can be quite confusing for other people. This is true for any other profession as it is for medicine. But whereas, not everyone wants to read about quantum mechanics; all of us need to know a thing or two about our health.

You will also notice in this book sections where I address the common medical myths you and I have been made to believe. I do this with the knowledge that most people make mistakes, or believe anything, not out of want, but out of lack of knowledge. But remember too, as you read my book, that medicine, just like any other profession, is a changing subject. What may be true today, may prove to be untrue tomorrow. However, the most important thing is to keep to evidence based knowledge. I have taken extreme care, believe me, to give you honest scientific views, as is prevailing at the present moment, and will therefore not apologize, where you to find such to be untrue tomorrow, with the discovery of more knowledge. This to my mind is the beauty of scientific thought. Needless to say, I have used only personal experience in all what you will read in this book. As I always say, I don't feel under any obligation to write something that in my mind does not coincide with what I consider as scientific fact, regardless of how many people may believe otherwise. I believe that evidence alone should be the guiding principle in any one's conclusion. That is just how science operates!

On the lighter side:

I should add also these thoughts about Doctors and Medicine; that

Medicine is the only profession that buries its mistakes!

- The doctor is the only male who you can beg to undress your wife and still pay for it! Jokes aside though, it's, an intriguing science, very wide and fathomless. So, in this book, I won't even pretend that you will read about all the conditions or diseases. That is not my intention. I set out to discuss with you some of the more common conditions you are likely to meet or have heard about, to correct some myths surrounding many conditions, to inform, to lay bare the fundaments of some diseases in the language you will easily relate to.

I have always thought doctors; a great doctor kills more people than a great general. For each illness doctors heal, if you look around, you will find they provide ten more diseases by reminding you and inoculating with the most dangerous virus of all, the idea that one is ill. No doctor is a good doctor who has not been ill himself!

Always remember that some remedies are worse than the disease itself and please know that nothing is more dangerous than a poor doctor, not even a poor employ or a poor childhood! Also remember that Dr. Diet, Dr No worry and Dr Play are the best doctors I have met!

Now sit up and enjoy the ride!

1. Your body is not stupid!

Whether you are asleep or awake, it's working all the time. Why it takes the trouble to keep you alive is somewhat of a puzzle...I mean why not just shut you up without any warning? Life is funny, it just wants to be .Its therefore surprising that we have people who still think the body is so stupid as to need detoxification by some healers or what we hear, to need colon cleansing!
For a religious person, this becomes somehow even more problematic, for ones runs the risk of thinking that one's Lord could have made an imperfect system, with no intrinsic properties to clean itself?
When you fart, pass urine, breathe out, or deposit a mass of some terribly smelly stuff in your toilet bowl, that my dear, is the surest cleansing machine, you can ever dream of! It takes a pretty amount of stupidity to think there is such a thing as colon cleansing or body detoxifying, as we see many charlatans claiming!
Your body is the most amazing machine to walk this earth, what with more than 100 000 000 000 000 cells in your brain alone, each ticking away every damn day of your life! Each knowing exactly what you need, each sending messages to the rest of the body day in day out, each churning away chemicals to regulate you!
Did you know that women tend to use less energy than men because of their generally smaller size? Did you know that your metabolism of breakup of foods go up each time you have fever, that high temperatures of the body raises the rate at which chemical reactions, metabolism or break up of foods? Did you know that for each degree of body

temperature above the normal of 36.6 degrees, you get 10 beats of increase in your heart rate?

When you understand that whatever you eat, be it carbohydrate, fats, proteins break down to give you energy eventually, that even your sweating from your skin is a way of controlling this beak down in energy? If you understand this it becomes easy to understand that problem of weight is mostly caused by our mouths! Excess food breaks to proteins, to fat and then ends up as adipose tissue! It therefore follows that adults who use more energy than they take in tend to use body reserves and therefore lose weight easily! You may recall when I wrote about control of weight I mentioned that I have never, you have never ever seen a fat prisoner! Do they take tablets or have a well-tailored regime to control their weight-no! All they do is to use (or are forced) more energy in terms of activity than what they take in. It's that simple! It therefore follows that thin individuals tend to have a high metabolic rate than fat individuals! Look at yourself, look at your child, if you are fat, or the child is fat, and just look at how you spend your day! Are you active? Is the child spending more time in front of the TV changing channels for cartoons, doing less running around, less walking, less playing?

Weight control =A+B

A=Food

B= Activity

Don't you swallow those tablets or drink those herbs in order to control your weight!

2. Basic understanding of common diseases

1.Infections-group of illnesses which have an organism, sometimes called germs as cause, usually the body reacts by a fever, such as
-bacterial-very small organisms which are often independent of the host, found in soil, on skin, in internal organs of the body like stomach, liver, bones, brain tissue, intestines or colons. Some organisms are sitting harmless in the body till appropriate changes make them virulent, or they may come from outside. Some really surprising ones like Helico bacter pyrori in stomach ulcers, a very good example of an infectious disease that was once thought the cause was acid!
-Viruses-even more minute things, some say, they aren't alive, as their lives are dependent on the host cell. These are the most stubborn to treat or cure (HIV, flu, Ebola, Zika, Hepatitis viruses, Polio, Small pox, Parvo in animals, avian in birds. No cure as such, mostly handled thru vaccines (special substances that produce defence cells that may destroy the virus or weaken it). Viruses are special, they are "dead' 'outside the host cell!
-caused by some other organism like malaria parasites

-Fungus-stuff resembling small mush rooms-cure is possible, Such as Cryptococcus, candida. Often found in the body or the environment, can live independently.

2. Cancers-Growths with uncontrollable direction, they feed on the host blood system. Causes varied from factors to direct causes like human papilloma viruses in cervical

cancer, or warts, radiation, unknown causes, genetically acquired. Difficult to cure as killing them often kills the very body we are trying to save! Some are easier to cure when found early such as prostate cancer, cervical, breast etc.

3 Psychiatric-Mind based disturbances. Often difficult to cure, others such as depression may cause other somatic (bodily) changes. Suicide may be thought as a psychiatric disease, badly handled, passion killings of spouses could as well be psych problems, not well recognized! Stress causes more bodily changes than anything else known!

4 Metabolic-illnesses such as diabetes, which happen when the body is not doing what it's supposed to well, the control mechanisms go berserk!

5 Genetic- You are born with it, you" can't" do much about it, such as sickle cell anaemia, cancers, metabolic problems, but infections are not under this group such as being born with TB! Some heart diseases fall into this category (some may be due to infections, or vascular, blood pressure related)

6. Idiopathic-largely unknown cause, like some cases of hypertension (high blood pressure), some cases of epilepsy

7 Pregnancy related- Such as preeclampsia, eclampsia, chorea.... these often disappear with delivery or within 6 weeks after delivery. Can be controlled

8 Vascular-Such as aneurysms (dilation of a blood vessels,), some form of strokes...may cause sudden death, varicose veins

So next time you may attribute cures to untrained hands or miracles... take a sip of water, and think!

3. Blood can tell a tale!

1. If it is darkish blue, you have poor oxygen in take

2 if its cherry red of normal consistency, there is adequate oxygen supply to your body

3. If it's watery, or too dilute, you probably are pregnant or have had too much fluid intake

4. Too thick and difficult to move, you have probably got too many red cells (a problem on itself!) or a cancer of the red cells.

5. Too many white cells (the normal being 4000-6000 per ml of blood-you probably have an infection with germs somewhere, and too much of the white cells, could be leukaemia, a form of cancer

6. Too few white cells, you probably have a viral infection or again some cancer-(leukopenia, aplastic anaemia) or your factory has folded or may be under extreme stress from some medications, herbal or conventional.

7. If your tongue or nail beds are pale white, you may have anaemia

8 if you bleed (or prolonged bleeding time) easily from any site, your clotting factors may be in a mess! Severe platelets (cells which help in clotting issues) depletion can lead to this as well

This is the bare minimum that a simple full blood count can show!

4. Read this!

There has been a few of us arguing about the origin of HIV, but with no medical training! Please note that every health worker when learning a new disease goes thru this process...
1.The definition
2.The cause, i.e. pathogenesis, the structure of the causative organism etc.
3. The various theories as to the origin from reputable sources (not face book!)! Epidemiology or spread patterns Worldwide and locally
4. What goes on in the body-Patho -physiology, Patho-anatomy-changes of the concerned tissue or organs under attack
5? The complications of the disease
6. Cure or treatment
7 Then the health worker keeps updating his knowledge as new info keeps emerging, discarding old ways and learning new things
So making us like we don't think at all and giving us what you get from face book as knowledge is rather foolish, sorry!

5. Family Planning

In my first book'' The Sceptic vol1, I loudly cried out of how pissed off I have been with some of our NGO's who have reduced reproductive health to advocating for condom placement in our primary and secondary schools. I wrote then that if you going to place condoms in my child's school, you might as well pack some condoms in the lunch boxes you give daily to your child; and I meant what I said, I stand by it even today, four years when I first wrote this! Family planning issues is not for pupils at Primary and Secondary schools, theirs should be books and books only! We don't send our children to schools to learn sex!
Jokes aside, what follows in this post is not for you the pupil or the student, it's for grownups!

When some of us were growing up, we were told only one thing, study and study the books! And we had few teenage pregnancies in our schools because our teachers and parents alike emphasized only moral training beyond anything else. I truly pray that this attitude is kept alive even today when we see the influences of weird western cultures in our schools, some of them perpetuated by the so-called NGO's, as they transplant strange cultures and teachings from across those with money to our schools, without taking into account local traditions and culture! Choosing is our everyday thing. We constantly have to make decisions on not only what to eat but on the size of our families-This is what we call *Family planning*, a deliberate decision on issues of family size, spacing of children and issues to do with timing when to have children.

It is also true, that was there a 100 % effective method of family planning, this write up would not be necessary. The plain truth is, there is none available! What often may work for you, may not work for me! A 100 % effective family planning method would entail total safety, inexpensive, readily available to those in need, with zero side effects and should be totally reversible, should not interfere with sexual feelings and acts. Such a method would not need a clinician to guide you. Such does not exist!

The simplest method known is the rhythm method, which depends on the character of the periods. In this method sex is avoided on the so called fertile days, which is usually the 14th day following the last period. Out of a hundred women, 20 will get pregnant using this method. In other words, we shall say that its failure rate is 20%. This is second only to no method at all, at failure rate of 70%!

Tying of tubes or tubal ligation, stands at a failure rate of 0.04%; vasectomy (when the male gets his tubes tied) at almost the same level.

The combined pill (oestrogen and progesterone) very popular among our women stands at 0.5% failure rate, the mini pill (with progesterone only) at 1%, is closely related to the injectables, the Depo Proveras. Then we have the various intra uterine devices or loops, at a failure rate of 1.5%, condoms at 2%, coitus interruptus (also

known as male withdrawal prior to full ejaculation) at 16 % failure rate. I won't even talk about the so-called morning after pill, because although popular among teenagers, no doctor or health worker can advise you to try it, it has a high failure rate!
When choosing which method to opt for it is advisable to see your clinician to see that you do not have inherent dangers within yourself and to discuss the various methods and their effectiveness of various methods available, for not only family planning but disease prevention as well.

6. To abort or not to, that is the question!

Most people when they hear the word "abortion" tend to think it is something that is "caused' the truth is abortion can be caused yes deliberately and sometimes it is just spontaneous (though rare!). Abortion is often induced one way or another.

What is abortion?

Loosely defined is the loss or termination of a pregnancy before the 24 weeks of gestation. Well at least in our Zambian conditions, this is correct, but in advanced nations the limit goes to 20 weeks. When I was a junior doctor, almost 30 yrs. ago, it was 28 weeks! Now anything between 24 -37 weeks is assumed viable outside the maternal environment, the womb (preterm pregnancy). Now allow me to cut out very detailed discussion in this post as it is not meant for medical people but the general public, and it is just one of the articles which will appear in my tenth book" ABC of health issues". So yes, abortion is loss of a foetus dead or alive before it has completed 24 weeks.

As I said in my opening remarks this can either be induced deliberately or spontaneous in nature. This reminds me sadly of thirty such cases committed in one of our secondary schools, I will not name here (I don't want to get lynched!) in the recent past just in one year! Sadly, these cases do not always end pleasantly even when medical personnel come in to try and save lives, some girls unfortunately kick the bucket trying to abort! This we shall call criminal abortion, as when it's done rather clandestinely, in very unhygienic environments, by people who cannot even tell the size of the uterus or womb! Now I mention this case simply because there is a section of very vocal religious groups who think medical abortions on request (as in RSA) is a sin and its murder! The truth is, whatever our attitudes may be, a girl (sometimes women) will always do whatever it takes to abort when the pregnancy is un expected, unplanned. By the way this includes the religious lot as well! And by the way, the foetus only developed a nervous system at around five months (in order to feel pain!). Most medical abortions are done when the foetus is not more than a group of cells, or sometimes very early when its organs are not formed, as such.

Those of us who have seen deaths of young women as a result of criminal abortions, will always preach that perhaps we as a country haven't done enough to prevent these unnecessary deaths. Family planning is readily available but young women are getting pregnant, and dying in doves! The 1972 law that permits abortion in our country when:

1. The girls or woman's health is threatened

2. When the foetus would be born grossly sick, grossly abnormal

3. When there is proven rape, incest, and defilement

4. There is extreme social distress by the mother to be (economic and social factors}

Have not am afraid helped to prevent the high rate of clandestine abortions leading to very terrible complications and sometimes death in the concerned population.

Abortions that a spontaneous are rare and can be caused by hormonal deficiencies, growths in wombs like fibroids, abnormalities of the wombs, intoxications from various drugs and general debility of the carrier, as regards her health, and sometimes we cannot really pin down the cause(idiopathic) or unknown aetiology. Miscarriage is another term I would like you to get straight. In our world, we talk of miscarriages a delivery out of whatever cause of a premature foetus or baby. Thus, we talk of miscarriage if a pregnancy is lost between the 24 to 37 weeks of pregnancy. As simple as that. Doctors will often call this kind of delivery as a pre-term delivery, which just means that before term!

Let us further for our confessions divide abortion into induced as in medically legal, medically illegal and criminal and hey I should say here out right that I have been in all of them at one time or another, some way. Don't you tell the cops, am being honest! If you meet a doctor who is not a nun or "father" and is going to swear that they never ever did the medically illegal one, he or she is possibly not being generous with the truth. I know doctors might kill me for this, but let truth be told!

Abortion really is some of form of continuum…its threatened, when the products of conception are intact and the external mouth of the womb is closed with a little pain and bleeding. Then you get the incomplete type when part of the products is expelled and part are the womb, then when everything goes out, it becomes a complete abortion. When the abortion will take place in spite of whatever, we call it inevitable, often the womb mouth is open in such cases, and the woman experiences a lot of pain and bleeding. My Cuban friends would call this kind of abortion "en-course", which to me is a piece of cake to decipher. Whereas, if the products of conception are trapped inside in a closed womb out let or cervix, with little or no bleeding, with a non-viable foetus, this is called a missed abortion.

Either of the above mentioned can be infected or septic. When a woman has more than two spontaneous abortions, we call it habitual, from the word habit.

Now I have laboured to explain these terms so you can have a good idea what really kills the women in abortions when they are carried out by unprofessional people. I remember as a junior doctor in the eighties doing daily more than twenty cleanings of girls' wombs following incomplete abortions. Most of these, if not all were clandestinely caused. Some of course died in compounds and villages before they could reach us for treatment. And we are talking of young lives here!

<u>Dangers of abortions</u>

Abortion if it's not carried out by trained hands is a killer. The immediate danger to an abortion is bleeding. Abortions does bleed, I tell you! If one escapes the bleeding, the next bomb shell to explode might be infection, mostly caused by use of dirty unsterile instruments introduced into the womb by unscrupulous individuals. The people who mess up with the anatomy of the woman without knowledge don't really understand that the rectum and intestines, and bladder are just like neighbours in there. The rectum is just behind the womb and the bladder just in front of it. So, it's not strange to get perforations or holes into the bladder and colons as pens or sticks are injudiciously pushed into the womb to commit abortions. Let us call these complications short term.

In the long run, a woman is bound to have further complications like blocked tubes resulting in infertility or sometimes the wombs neck gets loose leading to habitual abortions. Sometimes the infection is delayed and when it sets in tends to spread to the tummy or abdomen setting off a very dangerous state of infection involving the whole body, we call this, sepsis. This in turn can cause kidney or liver failure and you are on way to heaven uninvited! Was I writing this book for nurses or doctors specifically, I would have delved in how we manage abortions in medical facilities. But fortunately, or unfortunately this is not a medical book. So, let me quickly get to my point, suffice to say that the most frequent type of abortion, the incomplete one is treated by cleaning the womb of its contents. And we have recently developed clever methods where we can actually do this in the outpatient room, you get in and in ten minutes, you walk out!

You have heard the arguments! Abortion is murder, some claim. Others sing that abortion is killing human babies! Let me tell you this, abortion is in my view, dear reader is not murder, its termination of a pregnancy, not a human being! Of course, you would then challenge and say when does human life begin? Indeed, this question is not a simple one. The ovary or woman's egg is alive, we all know that, or should. The sperm of the male, those little clever speedy things in a male are also alive. Yet others would argue that life starts at conception. Like my catholic brothers. Whatever you say, a single cell is simply that a single cell, it's no more a human in my view, than the first brush stroke of a painting is picture or the first word of a book or novel. So, me for me, I would confess to you that I regard abortion as not murder but a prevention of babies from being born. In my mind allowing a woman to have full control of her body should be the aim of any nation. She is the best person best able to know what's best for her, not the parliamentarian, the priest nor the teacher not even I may add, the husband!

When I write this am aware this indeed is an emotive topic but what surprises me is that we often want to hear about abortions from our preachers or parliamentarians, people who have never ever seen a death directly related to abortions. If you want to find out what best an auto or manual gear box would surely ask the pope or the taxi driver? This is the tragedy of mankind. We have let decisions be made or lives by people who would do well to have their mouths closed! I will illustrate this point when I point out what the so called "pro-life" anti-abortions have peddled around. In fact, who is against life anyway? That they can only answer! The other extreme is as you have guessed right" pro-choice". Again, who really is against choice? The world never seems to stop amazing us, so let us use the two camps and see what they have

I recall at one meeting I was addressing on this topic to be told by one pro-life advocate that suppose I had been aborted, would I have liked it? This to me was a foolish attack for I simply answered that before I was born I had been dead all along and never suffered the slightest pain! In any case there're millions of paths life should traverse. Can we then argue that a woman who has had her menses had just thrown away a life? Or what about the millions of sperms you throw out in condoms aren't they potential lives or lives for that matter? So, this argument of destroying life just bounces off like a helium filled balloon!

The Bible and abortion

The Catholic Church that I grew under is very adamant about this. Abortion for whatever reason is a no- no affair. But if you take the Methodist or Presbyterian Church, they are essentially prochoice. It's another question if this difference in approach is based on any biblical teachings for in the book of Jeremiah Ch. 1 verse 5 its written, "before I formed thee in the belly, I knew thee and before thee cometh forth out of the womb I sanctified thee." While Exodus 20 verse13 is very explicit, "Thou shall not kill." Not sure though which killing is this, a bunch of unresponsive cells or a fully-fledged human? My medical training tells me that the foetus in the womb is not responsive to pain to about when its nervous system develops, about the fifth month! So am pre-empting those who say that abortion causes pain to the developing foetus!

 Bottom line is the scriptures cannot be used as a guide on whether we need to allow abortions or not for even slavery was allowed in the same book! I think we need to look elsewhere!

Look I grew up in the Catholic Church but reading the bible I have found in some areas it's got very powerful advice as in proverbs or Ecclesiastes but just look at the contradictions I have picked up before you throw it at me as authority:

Genesis 32 verse 20 says men have seen God while John 1 verse 18 writes that no one has seen God!

God does not keep anger forever –Jeremiah 3:12 and in Jeremiah 17:4 it says, God keeps anger forever.

Genesis 2:7 as well as Genesis 2:19 says, God creates man, then animals while just below this in Genesis 1:24 -27 it says God creates animals then man

James 5:16 says man can righteous and this is repeated in Genesis 7:1, Job 2:7, James 2:19, where as in Romans it says man can't be righteous

Mathew 20:29 writes two blind men healed on the road and Mark 10:46-47 says one blind man healed on the road

Its contradictions everywhere. Do people who use this book as a guide really read it attentively? I would not use such a contradictory document as a guide in such complex issues as abortion! For me it is not a religious question but a sexual reproductive question!

And in any case if God is the cause of everything, then even spontaneous abortions are caused by him. So, one would ask if he can do it, why can't we?

… Or like one of my naughty friends likes to say people resort to the bible to authenticate anything and everything because it's so much easier than things like logic, facts, evidence, science, common sense, proof, knowledge, confirmation. I find it a matter of when religion meets your moral standards, one tends to promote it so that fundamentalists, deceitful fundamentalist nut jobs can take advantage of the parts that seem to work for them and ignore other parts that seem to negate their deep held views. This is seen more glaring as regards the question of abortion. Like I like to point out many of these anti-abortion protagonists are find nothing contradictory in supporting death penalty!

What would you choose as a guide, a book written by sheep handlers more than 1000 yrs. ago, an inconsistent book, with mistakes not changed that has not been changed for a long time or a sober scientific look, where ideas are improved upon, mistakes fixed, and supported by modern thinkers? I go for the second option…

The bible scares the shit out of me and I wonder why one would use it as guide…check this…Mathew writes" If your eye makes you to stumble it is better to tear it out and throw it out-It is better for you to enter heaven with one eye that two eyes and be thrown into the lake of fire!" It doesn't become any scarier than this!

Arguments against abortion- Pro -life

1. Abortion is murder-this is the view of the mighty Catholic Church, headed by the Pope. It looks at the sanctity of life as non-negotiable. Not even it will result in the death of a mother carrying the baby!

2. No civilized society allows taking the life of another intentionally. To this one I ask, how about the death sentence?

3. Don't terminate, give out the baby for adoption. Not many women would risk their lives for another woman!

4. Do punish the perpetrator and not the baby. This again assumes the baby is responsive to pain at an earlier period. We have already dealt with this one, the nervous system in a late comer on the scene.

5. Why abort? Teach contraception and abstinence. This sounds good but the truth is the young people are doing it and dying in doves form criminal abortions

6. Never allow abortion because the young person especially does not know what they are doing. This too is a weak argument; they damn know exactly what they are doing! Not in this age of internet and Google!

Arguments for abortion-Pro-choice

1. The foetus does not feel pain, nor notice anything in the first trimester (first 13 weeks) of pregnancy. The foetus cannot exist independently outside the womb. It cannot lead a separate life

2. The women will still get pregnant and especially teenagers with increased maternal deaths related to criminal abortions. So why not offer them better options and prevent obvious unnecessary deaths?

3 Teenage pregnancies if allowed to term carries with it serious health risks

4.Some maternal conditions are not conducive to carrying a pregnancy to fruition such us heart problems or serious diabetes or kidney disease/Here the prolife will counter and say why get pregnant if you know your status? Now for me a medical practitioner, will tell you, the young people or some women don't just listen, they still will get pregnant!

5. Some social circumstances are a risk to a developing baby. Such as extreme poverty

6. Women cannot be forced to carry a pregnancy to fruition if it is as a result of incest, rape or defilement

 Arguments are many from both sides; here I have only scratched the surface. The truth however is that unwanted pregnancies will occur and criminal abortion will be carried out. Women will continue to die.

I have been at it in maternity care for over a quarter century now and I pretty remember every death of a teenage mother as a result of a criminally induced abortion. These deaths are unforgettable and they are painful! I remember a case of a sixteen-young lady who committed an abortion in one of the compounds, was admitted to our hospital with a distended painful tummy, with an open foul-smelling womb neck. We got to work on her immediately in theatre, having diagnosed a spread of infection with pus the abdomen. Our findings were gruesome, her small uterus or womb had been perforated with an instrument, it was partially rotten, and next to the womb the colon had multiple wounds as well. Well to save her life we had to take out the womb, and cut out a large section of the damaged colon, we then put her intestines though the abdominal wall just beside her navel for elimination of stool while her wound healed! She was sixteen! Oh yes, she was as well an anaesthetic risk as she had heart stoppage three times during surgery. We saved her minus her uterus at 16 yrs. of age! Sometimes in my quite moments I usually wonder what could have become with this young lady. Or can I forget my neighbour's child, a beautiful coloured young lady who took some traditional medicine that eventually took her life in my hands attending to her. Neither can I forget a beautiful young girl who took an over dose of chloroquine in order to procure an abortion. All these young souls died with me frantically trying to save them, most painful deaths. What most people don't know is that the womb is not directly connected with their mouths! Whatever you drink has to first go through your liver and blood to reach the womb!

Now when I advocate to give women rights to have a medically supervised termination, am saying this with the experience of the pain many of us and their relatives went and continue to go through. Many of the so called loud pro- life have never lost a life out of their hands during their lifetimes. They do not know how it feels or they pretend they do…especially form causes you know are preventable.

As for my good catholic church that brought me up I have the following questions:

1. Aren't the fathers, nuns, and brothers who stay without producing children, in a way denying the potential of life from promulgating? What is the difference between your sperms rotting in you, which are alive, and a few cells that are as result of conception? Of course, I can pretty guess their answer; life starts at conception! Really? May be not?

2. What do you honestly do with a woman who conceives out of rape, incest or a girl that conceives out of defilement?

3. What do you seriously do with a woman that conceives and has a medical condition, not compatible with pregnancy?

4. What about the teenagers who get pregnant, knowing that delivery carries a greater risk to these girls than a medical abortion?

5. How do you stop the ballooning maternal deaths out of clandestine abortions?

6 How do we marry the human rights of women to not allowing them to take full charge of their bodies?

7. What can we do to the fertilized eggs that are as a result of failed in vitro (outside human body or test tube) attempts at producing babies? Is this murder too, since they are thrown out into the bin?

The current law in Zambia demands that not less than two doctors must be satisfied that one of the conditions mentioned above are in order before one can have a medical abortion. Many girls and desperate women do not as a rule even try this route! Also, social distress has not been in my view been sold out to the women and girls for some reason by those whose job is to educate the masses! Is it because the Catholic Church, about the largest denomination in our country of 90% Christians has bulldozed us all in its refusal of abortion for whatever reason? Just like the Pope does not allow contraception of any type in his church regardless of the HIV epidemic! Africa, like the rest of the world is confused on the question of abortion. There are as you know 54, well with South Sudan now, let us say 55 countries in Africa. Each country has based on religious, ethical, political or social issues resolved this question their way. We can roughly separate the countries in three groups; those that have made it completely illegal to have an abortion for whatever reason, mostly Muslim countries, those who allow it if the woman's health is endangered like Zambia, Malawi, Tunisia and others and those like Republic of South Africa that allows abortion on demand.

When I was young medical student in the early 80, s in Communist Russia, I was impressed with Russia's liberal views on abortion. Any woman or girl who wanted a termination got one without any hullabooh, so it was with many Eastern countries then and am sure the situation is still the same today. Sometimes I have wondered if my liberal views towards the rights of women to take control of their bodies were as a result of this influence. I really do not think so. I have no doubt in my mind my gynaecological work and the deaths I have seen of young people, unnecessary deaths, could be the deciding factor that has swayed me to openly call for women to be granted full control over their bodies.

Zambia my own country has taken the middle road. Abortion is allowed following the 1972 abortion law only in certain circumstances, none of them social. Abortion in my country is allowed if the health of the woman to carry the pregnancy would be compromised, in cases of incest and rape. My problem with this position, dear reader stems from the fact that this decision was made more on religious lines and does not therefore really give the women the chance to fully utilize this service. Information is deliberately withheld prompting many a woman resorting to dangerous back street abortions, resulting in the country loosing unnecessary lives and spending almost the equivalent of 2, 5 million USD on treatment of abortion related complications a year. This situation cannot be allowed to continue like this!

The epitome of democracy, the USA, to which our politicians in Africa look for guidance is equally "confused" as each state has its own laws regarding abortion, disregarding the US supreme court's decision to have granted women full control of over their bodies. And this is America!

The Scandinavian countries in my view has the most progressive laws regarding abortion, with the UK, France, Germany coming a close second.

I don't know about you, but I think RSA, under Mandela then, established arguably the most progressive laws in Africa. They not only abolished the death penalty but they gave all women the right to abortion on demand, this as which was passed in1996 and became effective February 1997 saw a sudden decrease in maternal deaths related to unsafe abortions.

Elsewhere the situation is gloomy, like in the state of Chile, in South America, which is predominantly catholic and has under no circumstances allowed abortion, even if the life of a woman would be endangered! The only reason advanced is the sanctity of life. A very old argument I must say! And a loose one at that as the other side of the coin more lives are equally lost, talk of sanctity of life!

Does it occur to these nations denying women their rights that reproductive rights are no more different from issues of gender equality and freedoms? Making something illegal is not the same thing as making it not to happen.

Back street abortions will go ahead in the absence of a clear well thought about permission for women to take charge of their health. And the sooner the politician or priest gets out of the vaginas and concentrate on something more tangible, the better!

In Swaziland, the nation finds it perfectly alright to illegalize abortion but allows an excited young man, a king, to get a virgin girl each year of his rule as a wife! At the time am writing this (2015), the fellow has more than 15 young girls as wives. Are these not double standards on the part of the quiet religious leaders and politicians of that small nation?

Ugandans never made any noise when their President Idi Amin had taken 5 women as wives, had 30 mistresses and made 34 children. Now listen to the noise on gay rights and abortion, it's like an atomic bomb is about to be dropped on the nation! Africa cannot stop amazing you!

I had covered the issue of adoption as an option to abortion that we hear form the pro -lifers, but let me ask this, does these men suggesting this option ever think what it feels like to carry a pregnancy for a good nine months only to give away its product to someone who hasn't suffered for it? I say these men, mostly politicians and priests should learn to keep out of the doctor's office and off women's bodies. Let me end this chapter with something silly...

If you don't like gay marriage, don't get it

If you don't like cigarettes, don't smoke, for God's sake

If you don't like sex, don't do it

If you don't like porno, don't watch it

If you don't like alcohol, don't drink it

If you don't like guns, don't buy them

If you don't like abortion, don't have one

If you don't like your rights to be taken away, then don't take away someone else's, period!!

It beats me that we still should be fighting for the right to choose. Is it any body's business but he woman who is pregnant? The right to abortion in my view is part of a comprehensive health care package. What would you do to the 200 plus girls kidnapped by Nigerian Boko Haram and were found pregnant? To deny these young souls the right to termination would be tantamount to another kidnapping of their lives!

Is it not time that Zambia joined RSA and UK, Russia and many other advanced countries, in allowing women and girls to take charge of their bodies? Is it not time to allow abortion on demand? Should the parliamentarian or the churches, which have never ever seen the deaths in our facilities due to criminal abortions be the ones to decide this very important reproductive health question?

My young friend, Mweemba Sichilima, a former student of Hillcrest as well, after reading this puts up a few comments which I think you might enjoy:

"There is extreme social distress by the mother to be (economic and social factors}
that's a loaded one, and very open to any interpretation. Personal ordeals in the matter of people close to me lead me to believe that the final choice is best left to the Mother to be since it is a well-known fact that unplanned pregnancies have a bigger social implication on the mother than on the father.
The Father doesn't walk around with big fat load of the evidence of their mischief!
However, I think the father to be must be acquiescent, especially in helping to establish the "Social distress" factor, and also balancing out the responsibility of the pregnancy.
I know society has its ways of discouraging pre-marital sex and or unplanned pregnancy.
Our Society places all the financial responsibility of a pregnancy on the Father. Some tribes simply leave the woman at the man's house.
One would think the stigma is enough to stop us from running around having sex without protection. But alas it is not.
For you Doc, the medical part is pretty simple and you are a hundred percent right. But looking at our social and religious background, as well as protecting the sanctity of family... It's a tough call.
Parents have it tough, my brother. It's not really black and white. I am currently pondering, how do you play the balancing act between:

1. teaching children to be responsible when having sex is using protection, or even better, just ultimately reserving it for when they will have a lifelong partner ready to take on the responsibilities that it entails? "
2. teaching children that a child is a gift to be cherished, while at the same time teaching that abortion is a readily available escape route if you don't want to take responsibility?

I think you will be hard-pressed to find a group of individuals ready to pick up that banner in this country. Maybe a bunch of you Docs can do it. You have ample motivation for it.

I am most certain the nurses won't. Those guys seem to cherish the opportunity to stick it in the face of the patient that "This is what you get for being mischievous". Sometimes, even when they are dying!

7.   Concoctions for abortions

1.When you take water, any fluid or drug, it of course, goes into the stomach, then to the liver to be broken down or stored, then onto the kidneys thru blood... and lungs for expulsion.

2. Now anything passing the liver thru blood has to pass thru your heart, and then to the brain...and this is where the worst can happen! Depending on the strength you are likely to damage your brain cells (encephalopathy)...not to talk of the adverse effects on your liver and kidneys!

3. Then only does your medicine produce a toxicity on the womb thru blood, your womb may lose the contents, but not before you are too sick or almost dead!

4. Other means like introducing pens or other foreign objects have a direct danger of introducing infection or perforating the intestines which lie next to the womb. The infection can have immediate complications like spreading or can work way afterwards blocking your tubes (infertility). The other danger may be serious bleeding from the sudden detachment of harming of the inside walls of the womb!

Medicines can have multiple effects on the body, so it's not safe to take anything which has no selective action on the womb! This is the danger of all the strong teas, and other concoctions we hear about! Keep away!

Note: Medications used in hospitals and procedures for planned abortions take all this in cognizance! The doctors know the selective action of the drug being given, and they know the anatomy if instruments are used!

8. Masturbation-the truth!

First the basics of sexuality in man and woman...
Sex is a product of a fertile mind, it happens in the mind. Boys or men do have wet dreams in which they become erotically aroused in a dream and actually come off! This normally happens when a boy or man, who is sexually active, has had a big break before engaging in sex. The

body is clever, it has a way of self-cleansing using the subconscious mind. When a boy, girl, woman or man consciously brings oneself to orgasm thru different means, this is what is called masturbation (self-stimulation to orgasm). The satisfaction according to the body, the brain, is the same as the actual sexual act.

So then how does a normal sexual response become unhealthy? Unless of course in rare circumstances, the man or woman takes conscious steps to replace for good the mode of sexual gratification, and then want to change to the real act after a long time. Perhaps one could then talk of minor psychological difficulties, but such cases are as rare as snow in summer!

In few words masturbation has no dangers to health!

9. Let us talk epilepsy

...and only for the simple reason that often heath workers are said to know nothing about this pathology will be brief.

1. definition- loosely understand it as a tendency to have seizures or convulsions and I only address it because I hear a lot of people claiming that doctors cannot manage it...it has to be treated by traditional healers or pastors! Nothing can be further from the truth...so read on!!

2. Who can have it? Just about anybody can have fits or as we say seizures or convulsions. Statistically we know that one out of every twenty people will have had

fits at one time or another in their lives, however only about one in two hundred people will have repeated episodes. For some people, it may just be in child hood but for others this tendency to have seizures may continue well into adult hood

3.What causes seizures?

- Often no cause can be found. Not the same reason as saying there is any cause as most people assume, but our current knowledge may be limited! You can be apparently healthy individual, so to say, and still get seizures!! These kinds of epilepsy we sometimes call primary or idiopathic (not idiotic!). It appears that nature sometimes just places you among those with a higher propensity to get fits

- Sometimes we can find the cause-anything that damages the brain function can cause fits. Things like accidents to the head causing head injuries, strokes, brain infections like meningitis or malaria, encephalitis, or just previous difficult birth. Sometimes we find you may have tumours in the brain, sclerosis (understand as a hardening of some brain areas), or rarely so some inborn or genetic predisposition to fits.

4. Can you get it from inheritance? Here let us just say no and yes. Science has sometimes identified some genes responsible for seizures, but not always. Let us leave this one for another day!

5. Can you get it from another person? Certainly not!!

Now a bit of trouble for you, but will try to be simplistic!!

6. What's a seizure or fit or convulsion?
Well we all know the brain is the control centre for your body. It's made of up of millions of cells (that do not regenerate, hence stop abusing it with your boxing!!), these cells or neurons as scientists call them receive and transmit a hell of info from your body and surrounding. So if for some reason known or unknown these connections malfunction, the messages get disorganized and a seizure or fit may result. The types of fits you get will depend on the region of the brain affected.

7. Types of fits---loosely we can divide them into two main types-generalized or partial. Now if the seizure is generalized, it means the whole brain is affected by the malfunction, you end up losing conscientiousness or awareness, so to say. If you don't mind, let us call this type of fits tonic-clinic and absences...the French called them grand mal seizures
Partial or petit (small) mal let us call them focal seizures.

8. What happens--- in generalized fits, you lose consciousness, you may shit, or urinate, fall down, often with a loud cry, the body, the whole-body jerks uncontrollably, saliva may drip from your mouth (by the way eclamptic fits in pregnancy are one form of these major fits). After a few minutes the fits may subside, and you then enter into a short sleep before waking up. You may actually resume your normal work or activity after the fit

9. Absences-----here I think we all have heard of especially children just becoming suddenly blank, staring pointlessly

ahead or if they were writing they suddenly stop writing without reason, with a blank look. You can understand these types of seizures like day dreaming!! Fortunately, these are easily dwelt with by medical experts if a child is brought for their attention. The problem with us Zambians and Africans we think every Jim and jack knows it all, and we often take to *"Ngangas! "*Or even pastors!

9. Can you remain aware while having a seizure? Sure, you can, when only a small portion of your body is jerking or fitting. Won't go into details but sometimes we call these fits complex partial seizures. You really are aware of what is happening.

10. Triggers to epileptic fits vary-hunger, tiredness, fear, stress, or forgetting taking prescribed medications, sometimes strong lights like disco lights etc.

11. Auras--- are just warning sensations some people may get before fitting, not everyone may get them. But that's to them people well known with epilepsy can take measures to move away from dangerous situations before the major fitting sets in.

12. Treatment---Don't take the patient to chancers. Medical people can help you control seizures, even if they may really be no final treatment. The people who observed you fitting are interviewed and you may get a brain scan or a machine attached to you that registers the work of your brain...encephalograph or in full, EEG--- electroencephalography. Some children do grow out of

epilepsy while others may need medications to control fits. Sometimes if you don't fit for two or
more year's medications are carefully withheld. Sometimes surgery to remove a
portion of your brain if not big is done by Neuron - surgeons (remember Ben
Carson?)

13 Damage- if you don't injure yourself during a major episode, no damage
results to the heart or brain permanently. Unless of course yours is too frequent and too prolonged. Do not attempt to move a fitting person till the fits have stopped. Put them in a sideways position away from objects and wait!

14 working----you can do any work other than driving trains or planes, you can take part in any sport, but please make sure you are not alone when you decide to swim! Wear a helmet when cycling and avoid busy streets. You may drive a vehicle if you have no fits for more than two yrs.

15 Alcohol----please avoid it, though you may just be lucky enough to take in small doses, consult your doctor that the medications you are on is not in conflict with a bit of alcohol!!

16 Lastly don't stop medications without medical advice and if you are a woman you may get pregnant and deliver a normal child.
 Always consult your doctor and good luck, you don't have

go to the traditional healer, the African patient is so much excited over.

10. Meningitis

There are few diseases caused by germs which can turn fatal so quickly! Meningitis is one of them. Someone can die within a few hours of catching it.

What Is It? Meningitis simply means inflammation of the covers of the brain. You are aware that the brain is protected by the bones, the scalp bones and the vertebra bones; under them you will find some very thin covers whose function is to further caution the brain tissue from outside invaders and blows. Also between the blood vessels and the brain there is a barrier called the hematoma encephalic, which has to be breached for infection to get to the brain? Meaning not all germs or virus has the capacity to breach this barrier. This could be one of the reason the brain is such an important organ. As the body's CPU, it requires multiple defence systems. Cause of Meningitis 1. Bacterial-meningococcal, pneumococcal, tuberculosis and others 2. Viral-Most virus including flu viruses can cause meningitis 3-Funguses-As in Cryptococcal meningitis, common with HIV victims Symptoms the most common complaint is persistent throbbing headache which never gets relieved by such pain killers as parasols or aspirin. Confusion is also often noticed in such patients. Fever or increased body temperature is also noticed. Later you can have bulging of the fontanel as in kids (these are the deeps in the scalp bones), neck stiffness and spinal stiffness. Sometimes the patient develops seizures or fits of the body, all the way up to losing consciousness.

Diagnosis Talking of diagnosis perhaps here I should mention first the so called dreaded lumber puncture which most people accuse as cause of deaths of their patients. I should mention that this is just a needle prick at the lower back, about the level above below which the spinal cord ends. So just like any injection, it can and does carry a certain risk but not what most people think. Lumber puncture on its own, done by doctors with knowledge of anatomy, does not in self, kill the patient! What kills the patient is the disease itself, and I said when there is delay in treatment or is diagnosed late the dangers of dying are very high. We see most of our people in Zambia and Africa in general bringing patients rather very late to the hospital and then to make matter worse relatives start to waste more time quarrelling with health workers when a lumber puncture is planned to be taken. Thus, the patient is either brought late or the condition gets worse as relatives consult each other on the merits and demerits of the procedure! This is rather very unfortunate situation as doctors hate to do procedures without consent of the patient or their relative if unconscious. Medical ethics demand that no treatment should be forced upon any one. So, no, lumber puncture does not kill! A few drops of spinal fluid about 2 malls in each bottle is all that is required to carry out a biochemical and microscopic analysis, including determination of levels of sugar in the spinal fluid. All these are necessary for doctors to know what type of germ, virus or fungus is a causing the disease. Treatment is then specifically tailored towards the causative organism. Other investigations done can be an x- ray of the chest, a full blood count and a urine analysis. Sometimes a malaria slide is done to rule out malaria which can present with similar symptoms.

 Treatment largely depends on what is causing the meningitis. Most times antibiotics are given through the vein to try and treat the patient quickly. Untreated meningitis can lead to a quick death; a poorly treated case can result in the patient developing long term complications like paralysis or mental disturbance. Fungal meningitis can be treated for longer period even up to 6 months as in cryptococcal infection. In parting let me emphasize once more that do not fear a lumber puncture, it's safe and may save your patients life! This should take us to the lumber puncture myth you have all heard of.

11. Lumber Puncture myth!

We have all heard the cries" my sister or brother died shortly after the doctors had done a tap on her or him." Some relatives would kill a doctor if they found out he had done a lumber puncture on their patient. It's sad, but the information out there is misleading.

A lumber puncture is a procedure where by doctors take a small amount of fluid from your lower back and in good hands it only takes a single prick!

Doctors cannot carry out a procedure to kill your relative! Meningitis, that infection of the coverings of the brain if not treated in time is a killer. Causes can be viral. Bacterial (germs). Tuberculosis, fungal (often cryptococcal). The patient develops a severe headache up to loss of consciousness if left unchecked, some do fit or become confused. The tap of fluids is done in order to find out the cause of the meningitis, so that doctors may know exactly which drugs to use. The noise we hear about relatives dying is largely an exaggeration as people are often brought late to the medical facilities. It's not the tap that kills but the meningitis!!

My message is one, please take your relative to the health facility in time, the tap might just save their life!!

12.   Why HIV isn't a biological weapon!

1. It cuts across all nations, poor, and rich, some less affected than others but affected all the same.
2. A biological weapon would need to have some form of storage, such storage should not change the virility or strength of the weapon
3. Such a weapon has to have mass destructive tendencies in a short period of time to make any impact, not yrs.! HIV takes yrs. to develop into Aids, sometimes not even always!

4. The delivery weapon would not be thru sex mainly as the front line of fighting soldiers rarely engage in mass sexual acts! Neither can HIV be delivered thru a bomb!

5 A biological weapon to be effective must spread very fast and be difficult to stop or control. HIV is easily stopped by abstinence and use of condoms!

6. A weapon like that must be very difficult to trace. HIV is simple to diagnose!

7. A biological weapon such as anthrax germs and some nerve agents are known to stay long outside the body of a human or can easily spread thru the atmosphere...HIV when exposed outside the human blood (cell) does not survive more than 10 minutes at the most!
Please stop the conspiracy theories circulating that HIV is a weapon aimed at blacks! Hope you have listened!

13.   LIFE...How much do you know?

I see a lot of us don't want to read stuff and learn. Let us collect the little we can to make a bit of sense where there is so much confusion.

What is the purpose of life? How does it progress? Where do we really come from?

Science improves with time, many of these questions we really aren't sure, but ask them we must and look for answers we should encourage. Warning...this is not a religious discussion but a scientific one based on available knowledge. Facts are facts even if you don't agree with them!

LICHENS- these living things are the most surprising, they grow on rocks by producing acids that dissolve the minerals in rocks that this algae feed on. I mean who can eat a rock? You aren't the most amazing life form, the lichen is!

For this algae, which are living things to reach the size of a shirt button it takes 50 years! To reach the size of a dinner plate, it takes thousands of years. So, then you ask what the purpose of life is. Life my dear just is, it exists for its own sake, not for your sake! Life exists for itself!

Humans- Homo sapiens, four legged mammals, who think life has a point because these animals have plans, aspirations and desires. Therefore, life exists for these chaps! No way, and if you don't believe it, read on....

EARTH....Forget the stories Earth is really old, we know that, and you should know that as well! It's not

6 000 yrs. old please! It's a massive 4, 5 billion years or slightly more!! Don't ask me how we know this, that's the easier part of this story. We can even tell you how old you are to the second even within Zambian or any African facilities. So, let us not dwell on this one. So yes, the earth is 4.5 billion years old.

Early life...However it started, no one can really say but we are pretty sure man has not always been on this earth this long. It was a world of micro-organisms that first appeared in the waters, and then came sea plants, then jelly fish, then the plants got onto the barren earth and we were on our way!

On land first appeared insects which eventually had to be winged in order to escape and survive, then came the dinosaurs which following some meteoric impact with earth quickly disappeared. Just pray some large rock from outer space does not crash into your town soon, because we all shall be history! (As matter of fact, one such rock is approaching our earth! Hope it misses us, as scientists predict, so don't you start shedding tears!!}

Yeah, so followed other mammals and then we chaps emerged, probably just close to 3 million yrs. ago, we aren't so sure (Early man started in Africa, if you have forgotten}
Just so you don't think, you have always been here, species on earth do routinely crumble and disappear either out of global warming, global cooling, changing sea levels, oxygen depletion, epidemics or diseases, methane

gas leaks from the bottom of the seas, meteor /comet impacts, volcanic eruptions, sonar flares. So, you see, it's a dangerous ride around the sun, though it's free!!

To sober you up a bit, it's not a secret now to say that 99.9% of all early species are no longer with us! Any species, for your information, lasts about 4000 000 yrs. on average on earth and hey we are just reached that---but I am not watch tower follower to tell you, the end is tomorrow. With our madness, it could have been yesterday!!

Dinosaurs- Some fanatics think these animals never ever were there. We have enough proof they all kicked the bucket when a massive impact hit the earth with the force of 100 million mega tons, enough to have killed the present 7 billion people, a billion times over! Amazing is it not? Fossils don't cheat! The acid rain that followed wiped out a lot of other species, fortunately we hadn't been around, you see! Only the water based creatures survived to a certain level because of the calming and protective effect of the waters. Even the Zambezi crocs made it! And the stubborn lizards!

Why the drama?
To survive animals had to adapt quickly to escape predators in the waters and on surface and to the changing environment. With Mr Shark having emerged, many guys ran off out of the waters just to make it! The only thing was to develop the ability to get oxygen straight from the atmosphere instead of from the waters, but the chaps learnt quickly. You either learn or you

disappear! Here in lies the genius of Charles Darwin to have unravelled this mystery of life progression. Your job and mine now is to find out from where it all came from. It needs hard work and just prayers won't do!!

Can we start reading before we open our mouths, please?

And if you are ready for some more basic facts, read on.... *It's as simple as simple as ABC!*

14. DNA made simple

- stands for deoxyribonucleic acid
- It's the stuff of life
-its inside the nucleus in the animal cell, inside chromosomes
-it carries the instructions that make you
- For me I take it as the most extra ordinary molecule ever found!

- There is about 2 meters in every cell, resulting in something like 3, 2 billion letters of coding, giving you not less than 1x3 billion zeros of combinations. That's why no one has a voice exactly like yours!! Not even your twin!!

- You have about 10 000 million or 10 trillion cells inside you, that DNA inside can reach the moon and back many time (remember the moon is 386 000 miles away!}

-that's 20 000km of DNA inside you!

You know when it was all discovered? Not very long ago, just in 1869 by Swiss scientist, Johann Friedrich Miescher, who incidentally you didn't not give any Nobel Prize to, because it took ages for us to appreciate what this guy had unearthed! We can be so mean at times!

- All your proteins are made by its "'say" through RNA, which you may recall is some form of interpreter.

-----Surprisingly, DNA has only four chemical components which we all learnt in our biology class namely ADENINE, GUANINE, CYTOSINE, THIAMINE....Remember?

--- What we were not told is that 97% of this DNA is just junk, imagine!
----Now then what are genes you may ask? Good question! Take that genes are just instructions to make proteins, meaning, the so called human genome means just a text book, and genes are the pages to make the book, clear?
---Meaning the letter in the book, the genetic book, the genetic Alphabets are the sweet chemicals I mentioned earlier. Adenine, Guanine, Cytosine, and Thiamine
---And guess what, these fellows are arranged in a double Helix G-C
T-A

Now you understand why there can be so many combinations, I hope!

The other day, you were asking what the purpose of life is. Ha ha ha, you humans, DNA does not really care about you, it exists for its self, to perpetuate itself, stupid fellow! Life just wants to be. Perhaps you now understand why the instinct to mate is the most powerful of all instincts on earth and in life (am not sure what homos will say about this!}

Now if you thought you were special, get this, your DNA is 90% like that of mice, seriously! In fact, even grass shares about 35000 genes with you guys, humans! Are you sobering up now?

15. Your cells

Thank your cells!
1. Your cells that make you are 10 000 000 000 000, or ten trillion in number, an enormous number, you must say. This all started with a single union of a little guy, the sperm, 85 000 times smaller than the egg colliding together, and you were on way to you!

2. These little fellows are really metropolises and refineries at the same time. They are cities because they have everything within them, all doing different things, some sending messages, some removing rubbish, some cleaning up after you, some storing your foods, some defending you from your foes from within and from without. These guys are indeed little refineries, for without them, you would drown in your own poisons. The liver cells which live a lot yrs. do this for you, the brain

cells that live forever, since birth, are your central processing units, the commander in chiefs.... We should be thanking these little chaps for our existence, yet we go on with our daily lives without even noticing what they are doing for us. Sometimes we would rather go to lengths thanking some obscure creator far devoid of our experiences! Thankless you!

3. That fellow, Robert Hooke, we owe him a lot, he was the first person to describe a cell. By the way, do you know that your cell is really an electricity station? Yes, it produces electricity, though on minute levels so you don't get shocked, but plenty of it to make you feel it. When you feel warm, it is the electricity produced from your food and oxygen that you really are feeling. It's produced in what we call, the mitochondria, which is the power station of your cells. In here, your food and oxygen, as I said earlier, is converted into electric energy---So you have your own Kariba power station that never load sheds you, see!

4. Take your blood, which really is just a bunch of white cells and red cells in water. Thanks to it, you   receive about 8000 litres of blood getting to nourish your cells from your heart each day. In a yr. that is a whopping 3 000 000 of blood rushing to your cells! If you can't imagine how massive this is, take the Lusaka Olympic pool and feel it to four times its size. Surely these little fellows need plenty of nourishing!!

5. Everyone has heard of cancer, of course, which is the main reason am writing this thank you note. Your cells

really sometimes get confused, bombarded by quite a lot of foreign matter, they die, they fight, and sometimes they can die for you, but sometimes some rogue cell just loses it and keeps growing and growing without stopping, without any particular programme, this we call cancer cells. To tell you the truth, cancer cells are all the time happening and you don't even know it, because your white cells just doesn't tolerate stupidity and only they when fail do you really land in trouble. That's why some clever viruses, like HIV, would rather not mess up with your cells early, they hide and only appear when the good cells have been duped to think all is well inside. Hence, the difficulties at finding a cure for HIV.

Come to think of it, your body is the best doctor there is, the rest of us are just pretenders!! But now, can we thank our cells for once, pal?

16. HIV /AIDS…The current status…

Viruses are damn difficult chaps. Up to now the world has some 1000 or so flu viruses, and no cure at all! What makes them so stubborn is that unlike bacteria or germs, they are assumed dead and alive at the same time. Meaning they are only active when in host cells, or in some other living organism. Viruses are damn clever at dodging our medications, our natural defence cells, through mutation or other means!

Every Dec 1, is world's AIDS day. It's now almost three decades after the first cases and the world is still not found a cure for it! We have defeated small pox, another virus that killed thousands of people, in olden times. We have done this thru vaccination, not cure!

A vaccine is a substance that contains anti bodies or that initiates creation of defence cells of the body, it's no treatment. It's a preventative tactic, meaning those already with the virus cannot get any benefit, only those without.

However the world has been working at finding a cure, it's just that it's no walk in the park. As for all humans, we are all either infected or affected. There is no one who can possibly claim immunity from this disease, one way or the other. We have been affected by getting infected, or looking after our sick relatives, losing our relatives, losing productivity at work through missing work or being on numerous sick leaves. Only a fool can say in his heart he or she has never been affected or infected!
But sadly enough, some of our people through misguided pride have been thinking treatment for HIV can just be stumbled upon just like that, by people who can hardly hold the microscope the right way up! We waste valuable time and resources doing unwarranted studies, quarrelling, instead of arming our laboratories to do serious work, we waste time expecting miracles from prophets and pastors, instead of investing our moneys in scientists to work more productively. Even our African parliamentarians think they all understand the behaviour of HIV virus, when they don't! They should involve themselves in more productive debates that promulgating wrongly placed national pride on unworkable treatments!

To this group of miserable claims belongs the Sondashi formula, promulgated by one silly old man, a Dr. of constitution law in Zambia.

We must appreciate efforts of RSA, a country that gets 1000 infections of HIV in a day and has more than 7 000 000 people on therapy and the efforts it is putting into research for treatment and finding a vaccine for HIV.

Zambia has 700 000 people on treatment currently but we need to cover 1200 000 infected people. Unfortunately, most of our efforts have been primed towards building grandiose million-kwacha prayer houses instead of arming our research fellows at Tropical Disease Research Centre at Ndola! We somehow think you can fast or pray yourself to clearing HIV from the blood stream! Nothing wrong with praying, so long you put your prayers into perspective! Viruses listen to no prayers! Former President of Botswana Festus Mogae, a bull dog politician in the fight against HIV, adopted" routine test and treat" way back in 2003. What we in Zambia are just being informed, we are about to implement now. This approach is an opt- out, opt- in type, with immediate offering of treatment to the affected. In Zambia, we love somehow to move slowly sometimes! We also love to ostracize those who always caution us to ignore the" miracle doers ". We are also a nation that loves talking about nothing, elevating and giving prominence to guessers and traditional healers (and sometimes lawyers!) In very delicate disease entities. We somehow feel we are a nation on the move! Unfortunately, though, viruses have no respect to misplaced national pride. Viruses need large investments in laboratories; viruses are not politicians!

The South African vaccine research results won't be in for another three years, but we are hopeful that the vaccine trials may finally go above the required 50%-60% effectiveness or efficacy.

In combating disease, fasting and prayers aren't the way; you have to put money where your mouth is! One more thing though, just say whatever you like, Zambia won't discover the cure or vaccine for HIV, till Joseph's child returns from his heavenly holiday! This I am sure about!

Heart and You

Know About the Modern Killer Disease

No, you are wrong, it's not HIV/AIDS, and it's your heart! The heart attack is the new kid on the block and it's all because of us, our life styles. In the western world, it accounts for more than 70% of deaths, and in our developing countries its fast catching up as we join the sedentary life styles of the modern age.

You have obviously all heard the saying, "I have love for you in my heart. "The heart which is the central piece in poetry has no love in it, it's just a pump for your blood! It is equipped to send oxygenated blood to itself and the whole body. This heart which is the size of clenched man's fist is situated between your two lungs in the left side of your body. It has no love in it except four chambers, two chambers that collect blood from your body we call atria and two other chambers which pump blood to the rest of your body, we call ventricles. The two parts of the heart are separated by a membrane and some valves which regulate entry and departure of blood. The right ventricle sends blood to your lungs and the left ventricle to the rest of your body, and the left is therefore twice as thick as the right in muscle mass.

But first let us discuss the basics. Your heart beat is on average about 60-90 beats per minute, that's for an average adult. In fact, the bigger your body is, the slower is your heart beat. The bigger the organism is, the slower is the heart beat. Meaning that a day-old child has a normal heart beat of between 120-140 beats per minute, which drops as its body picks up mass. The elephant has 25 beats per minute, rabbits about the same as human babies; the mouse is 125 beats per minute. Am sure my cousins in the Eastern province of Zambia do not know that the mice they love so much have similar heart beats as day old babies!

A few things we do can however increase our heart beats. Coffee, going up stairs, sex, worry, and a sumptuous lunch, all increase human heart beats. Does the heart rest? Yes it does, and that is during each beat, its self-serving sort of job, automatic. The heart being like any organ in the body also does require its own blood supplying, in fact all organs do! It not only pumps the blood to each organ but is itself getting its own independent supply from two lines we call coronaries. Corona- from the Latin word corona which means crown or surround. Now you understand this is where we have problems-coronary heart disease or CHD, is all dependent on your life style. Our diet full of fats, cholesterol is killing us. Our daily stresses, which we face as we solve our daily problems is killing us, our increased blood pressure and high sugar levels is killing us. And sometimes just our heredity may be the time bomb that will eventually result in an early death.

To understand how our diet kills, you got to know a bit about the chemical produced in the liver from the proteins we take we call fibrinogen, This is what lies at the bottom of our problems as it is the one responsible for production of fibrin, a clotting agent, which helps us in arresting bleeding which may occur from time to time in our bodies.

Fibrin forms clots and these clots which can go anywhere, most importantly can become more dangerous when it clogs the blood supply in our own hearts. What increases the levels of fibrin? We have here smoking, increased blood pressure, fats, increased sugars in our bodies, age and heredity. So, any disposition of fats in the small vessels of the heart called coronaries is a dangerous undertaking! It results in a condition we call atherosclerosis, which is another clever way of saying your arteries have fat in them! The heart suffers! Depending on the extent of blockage you may suffer heart attack and die after four hours or shortly after wards, without warning, or simply fall down dead in an instant. This is the reason why many people appearing healthy on the outside can just suddenly fall and die! Some of our poorly informed African people will explain this as manifestations of demons or witchcraft!

You all remember Elvis Presley who died at the tender age of 42. But do you know what? On Post Mortem, his heart was found to be like that of an 80 yr. old man! Elvis Presley had very poor life styles and very bad diet!

Now here is what you do to control your cholesterol and fats to avoid sudden heart deaths:

1. Reduce levels of your stress- Stress causes the adrenal glands, small little organs on top of your kidneys, to produce high levels cortico- steroids which may make your heart to over work.

2. Reduce or stop smoking-Nicotine contained in your cigarettes is poison to your heart and brain cells

3. Reduce your weight-overweight people produce more fats in their bodies

4. Control increased blood pressure by diet or prescribed drugs

5. Reduce your intake of eggs to maximum of 1 or 2 per week

6. Use skimmed milk

7. Eat less cheese

8. Trim fats from chickens and meats before cooking

9. Increase your activity levels

10. Reduce on or stop alcohol consumption

Please note: We haven't here said go to the prophets for treatment or try to swallow some fancy tablets

BUT:

-Use vegetable oils in cooking, (like olive oil-I know it's expensive, but come to think of it, sickness is more expensive!)

-Use poly saturated margarines in frying and baking
-Increase your intake of beans and vegetables (don't overcook the veggies!)
-Increase your intake of fresh fruits, grains like oats
-You may also try to avoid use of contraceptive pills (they are bound to increase your bad cholesterol)
Again don't drive to your toilet, walk!

18.   Alcohol, the facts

Head-It's indeed a stimulant in mild doses but in higher doses is a suppressant. Alcohol is poisonous to brain cells that do not regenerate when they are killed. You have about 100 000 000 000 000 brain cells all in all, maybe that's why you sometimes don't see the damage. Alcohol is a drug, it's addictive; meaning it creates strong craving with repeated over use, and more and higher doses are demanded by the body as use rises. Users become more and more careless to self and responsibilities to care for family drops. Higher doses may result in complete shutdown of the brain activity leading to death.

Chest-The heart muscles suffers, as the heart may become dilated created a cardiomyopathy, which is another way of saying the heart's contractual powers are decreased as it dilates. Consequently, if the heart cannot pump blood effectively, then the lungs in turn become congested, oedematous or swollen with fluids, you drown in your own fluids! Oxygen supply suffers to the rest of the body and every organ suffers!

Abdomen-The stomach gets hit first producing vomiting as it fights back, eventually it may become inflamed producing gastritis, all the way up to over production of hydrochloric acid and other juices which may eventually cause ulcers or stomach cancer. Then your liver suffers. The liver cells start dying in -mass, as they get poisoned producing inflammation or hepatitis, all the way up to total shrinkage; we call cirrhosis, a condition that is not reversible. Sometimes cancer may develop, hepatoma as it is called. The early signs of damage to liver cells may be that you develop yellow eyes or jaundice, which itself is a toxin on its own right. The ability of the liver to detoxify your blood plummets flooding the body with unrequited toxic waste. The pancreas a small organ near your stomach that regulates your body sugars through production of insulin and helps in digestion by producing pancreatic juice, may inflame, producing pancreatitis or may become cancerous. Your tummy becomes painful and bigger!

Blood- Your body's production of blood cells suffers as ingredients from the liver for the production of blood cells such as erythropoietin and vitamins get depleted. You may develop anaemia or low levels of blood

Blood vessels- dilate or become bigger under the influence of the toxic effects of alcohol. Your blood pressure drops, oxygen transport to various organs suffers, your organs suffer!

Nerves- Your nerves become more and more paralyzed, penile erections may drop. Frigidity in women may develop. Alcohol as Shakespeare once wrote creates desire but takes away the performance! It is not true that alcohol actually improves sexual performance! Dead nerves don't perform well! Even appetite for food eventually wanes. Driving reactions gets impaired, judgment is messed up, encourages speeding as it gives wrong courage. Common inhibitions break down; our behaviours may become unusual and uncoordinated.

Pregnancy-Alcohol may induce abortions, premature deliveries, may result in brain affected babies at birth.

Increased alcohol consumption is a major public health issue of our times. Why then is there so much alcohol in the shops, you might rightly ask?

19. Stress Kills that Is If You Allow It!

We all have stress! I know of no man without one, the teachers have it, the doctors, the casual workers, the politicians, the president, your wife, girlfriend, your hubby, your boyfriend, the prophets, the Pope- Everybody!

Let us loosely understand it as nothing more than a non-specific response of your body to any demand made upon it. Thing is, in this modern world we all have varying demands. True we all react to stress differently, some too seriously, some easily. And that's where the major difference lies! Stress tries to prepare us to avoid the threat to our lives but it can also kill us in the process, if we don't take proper stock of it.

You have all heard of people who have suddenly collapsed and died after hearing bad news. You have heard of people admitted in hospitals following bad news or bereavements. You have heard of people committing suicides or attempting to do so after love affairs end; you have heard of people who end up in counselling sessions after love affairs have ended, after divorces, after losing monies in gambling scams.

If you are alive you have emotions, which is nothing but anger, anxiety, feelings of boredom, distrust, fears, frustrations, guilt, resentment, impatience, self-pity, and so on. All these are under the influence of our state of our minds. And our states of mind are in turn influenced by levels of active chemicals we release un- wittingly within our bodies, such as adrenalin, no-adrenalin. Depending on the levels of these chemicals and their influence on our bodies we may experience diseases or altered state of our bodies. Remember adrenalin is produced in some little organs above both your kidneys, called adrenal glands. These glands in turn are under the control of one small pear-shaped organ in your head we call pituitary gland or hypophysis which picks up cues from the brain and surrounding. Even menses if you are a woman can be influenced by the state of your mind by the work of this organ releasing or with holding chemicals to your ovaries!

Perhaps that is why you heard that during the Gulf war, some women developed absence of menses or amenorrhea as we call it in gynae practice. The mind is a mine field!

Your stomach may develop high levels of acids, all the way to being inflamed or ulcerated, you may have diarrhoea, your joints may pain and get inflamed(arthritis), you may have sleepiness or develop insomnia, you may experience panic attacks, your heart beats may quicken, your blood pressure may rise up, your breathing may be faster than usual. Practically any organ may suffer!

This should make you understand the apparent success rates of so called prophets who may claim to cure your conditions! Indeed, they some do, all because the mind is the cause of the disease though it may appear physical! Clutches may be thrown away; limping people may start to walk straight! So, called demon possessed, which is just a state of mild psychiatric disturbances may get healed! We only differ at explanations why such occur; they think its miracles while we know it's all in your doing unconsciously or consciously. These are not miracles!

What is the way out?

First get a physical examination from health personnel to rule out conditions that may really be there in the body, conditions that may be caused by viruses, bacteria, infections and other altered metabolic states like diabetes and blood pressure, cancers etc. . . . .etc. This will relax your mind.

Do not opt to run to alcohol or cigarette smoking, these things do not in the final analysis remove the problem. Avoid drug and herbal escape route.

This is where you need to use the well-known serenity prayer that states, 'God grant me the serenity to accept what I can't change, the courage to change that which I can and the wisdom to know the difference."

This to me is the most powerful prayer one can have! This is about the only prayer that really works!

Then think of one thing at a time. A cat that attempts to catch two mice at the same time, they say often goes hungry! Be flexible but focused, avoid procrastination, do not put unrealistic goals upfront to yourself, include leisure in your schedule, work, and develop patience. You see someone says that death is the ultimate relaxation developed by the body for us. Learn to take life easy! Relax! Have enough sleep, rest enough. If all these fails ask for counselling from qualified health personnel. Above all else don't forget to have some humour in your life. It has been proven that humour alone may help keep your hearts speed down, and may help keep your adrenalin release down. Do not take life too seriously!

Don't let stress kill you! Take the distress out of stress!

20. Miracle Foods?

In Zambia, today and in Africa in general you see a lot of media adverts about miracle foods, miracle drinks, miracle tablets, and miracle herbs to keep one healthy, to control one's weight to control cholesterol and so on. But do we really have such?

I have had my own relatives try to convince me that taking garlic, taking lemon drinks is that panacea to weight control and disease avoidance. Some have opted to take high sounding herbal concoctions as treatments. Some opt to eat only brown bread, take brown sugar, oats, and legumes as a control for cholesterol. Yes, these brown things may have a higher fibre content but believe me, it takes much more than taking 'browns'' to control weight or cholesterol. Perhaps, what many people are taking as what is working is that these things are incorporated in some other sensible diets and active life styles they may be having! Something low in fats, we should caution you is not necessarily low in cholesterol! I have written about this before, the only way to a healthy body is nothing to do with taking herbs or tablets but taking a varied array of foods, with plenty of veggies and fruits, taking foods in controlled amounts, not missing meals, and always being active in whatever you are doing. Live an active life style, avoid junk foods, and do not drive as, I always say, to the toilet! Walk!

21. Do you snore at night?

If you don't, you are lucky, but sleeping next to someone who snores can sometimes mess up your nights like a single mosquito can.

Have you noticed that this is a condition most prevalent among male adults? The snorer is mostly often being an older male.

It is said that the cause of this irritating condition lies in muscle relaxation of the intrinsic tongue and soft palate (the palate is the back door to your mouth). The tongue and the palate falls down upon your throat making it more and more difficult to breathe, hence the noise. Alcohol and tranquilizers like Valium taking before one settles to sleep tends to worsen the situation.

I remember my Chibuku loving late father being a terrible snorer during my village life. Having died when I was hardly 10 yrs. old I can't really recall his face but I can very well remember his hard snoring each time he came back drunk! It's a memory I have cherished a lot about my old man! He really had a way to upset my mother and the rest of us after each night he enjoyed his opaque beer! We all slept in small two roomed thatched huts!

Wrong posture is also perhaps the cause of a falling tongue in drunks as they sleep sometimes facing upwards. Obesity is another well-defined cause. Air way obstructive lesions may also be a cause for snoring especially in kids.

Snoring can more often than not result in sleep deprivation, hyper somnolence (affinity to sleepiness in the day), or sometimes can result in periods of apnoea or temporarily stoppage of breathing.

Here is what you can do to alleviate snoring:

1. Avoid drugs such as Valium before you hit your bed

2. Try to sleep on one side, left or right instead of with your face looking upwards were possible.

3. Reduce your weight

4. If you are next to the snorer jab them in the ribs, this can lead them to enter into lighter mode of sleep reducing snoring

5. If your child has adenoids or growths in the air way have them surgically removed. Avulo palate- pharingo plasty operation may help in severe cases.

6. Sometimes the scarring that follows a tonsillectomy may help the snorer, surgery on the tonsils tends to stiffen the palate as the scar hardens

22. Sugar is not the problem!

You have heard it all'' *Do not take too much sugar, you may get sugar disease!"* How wrong!

Well not completely wrong but almost wrong, yes! Sugar does not cause sugar disease! Sugar may worsen your sugar disease! Confusing? I hope not! But first let me tell you a little about what happens with the food we all eat.

We all need sugar. Sugar provides the energy for our cells to function, from brain cells, liver, lung, skin to literally every cell in the body. Without sugar the mitochondria which is the energy factory of the cells would be defunct. We all get sugar from two sources, from our foods and from our stores in the body. The liver stores sugar in form of glycogen after getting it from the digested food from our stomachs. There is always sugar flowing in our blood stream. Let us call this glucose. The regulation of which is under a hormone called insulin. Insulin, discovered in 1920, is produced in a pale-yellow organ near the stomach, we call pancreas; the same organ which produces pancreatic fluid for digestion of food. Insulin therefore regulates the levels of sugar in our bodies and it's up take into various cells in the body.

The Pancreas may insufficiently function due to many reasons. It could be a hereditary condition, or it could become inflamed or attacked by toxins, including alcohol, viruses or bacteria.

We commonly differentiate two types of sugar disease; Type 1, which commonly afflicts the young and type 2, which is often found in adults.

When sugar is high in the blood vessels it creates high osmotic pressure, which in turn leads to the pooling of water from surrounding cells, leading to dehydration. The kidneys jump in, they try to push out as much water as possible and often they may be over whelmed, leading to kidney failure. As a result of these high levels of sugar in the vessels a triad of symptoms is produced:

1. Polydipsia- Increased thirsty and drinking

2. Polyphagia- increase swallowing or eating

3. Polyuria-increased release of urine

All organs in the body as a result may suffer. You may develop poor eyesight, poor heart function, poor liver function, increased blood pressure, the skin may develop infections in form of itchy rashes or fungal infections, the vagina may develop increase discharges, abscesses may form in different areas and wound may take long to heal. One may develop strokes in the brain as well. All the way to losing consciousness or what we call coma.

What can you do if you are diabetic?

-reduce weight

- reduce intake of sugars and salts, as well as fats

-Increase your intake of veggies and fruits

-Increase your exercise levels-make sure that you don't exercise only when group of muscles in the body-chewing muscles!

-Have monthly monitoring of your sugars in the blood

-Avoid over use of cigarettes and alcohol

23. Pimples and Acne

Pimples is a condition that though does not kill but can be very stubborn to get rid of. This is a form of rash, a result of clogged pores in your skin, that part which forms the sweating glands. Fat is trapped forming round small masses. We often see pimples in the young age about the puberty stage when the hormones start to wreak havoc in the maturing body. Sometimes though, even dandruff on the head can cause pimples. Those women taking hormonal pills for prevention of pregnancy can also sometimes suffer from pimples. Surprisingly though, most people do not know that you can also get pimples as a result of having digestive problems! Not only that but even excessive stress can lead one to develop pimples, so can the action of some hair products as well.

When pimples are flat in appearance, this is what is called acne.

Causes of acne/pimples

-digestive problems

-liver and kidney problems

-respiratory or breathing problems

-High blood pressure

--stress

-hormonal effects

-bacteria and infections of the skin

-Allergy of some sort can also cause sometimes acne.
What is true for pimples is thru for acne! Now you can see
from above list while acne and pimples can sometimes
present very difficult issues as regard identification of the
real cause. The causes are numerous. The only thing to
emphasize is that acne or pimples never really killed a
man!

What can you do to reduce the likelihood of developing
pimples or acne? Well sometimes, sorry to say nothing!
You remember we mentioned earlier of the hormonal
changes that may take place in the maturing young
person. Sometimes acne can improve when along course
of antibiotics is used, in the form of oral medications, such
as the tetracyclines or the long acting twice a day, called
doxycycline. But this is only true if there is infection of
bacteria or germs on the skin. What is disturbing is such
antibiotics are supposed to be swallowed over a long
period, with antecedent problems this alone can cause on
the body of the sufferer such as prolonged diarrhoea,

rash, allergies and of course development of resistance to a given antibiotic. Am aware some of my colleagues resort to use of hydrocortisone or beclomethasone skin ointments on the patients. However, such approaches are frowned upon nowadays as ill conceived, as the side effects can sometimes outweigh the benefits (, inflammation of the stomach or even stomach ulcers, high blood pressure, promotion of low immunity...)

Try this:

Use cleansing, toning moisturizers as such are largely harmless. Try to use lavender oils, apple cider and even lemon juice cider application may help, vinegar may also assist. Lemon juice contains vitamin c that helps in skin healing. Zinc Sulphate, 36 fatty acids preparations may also help. Tomato juice applied overnight on the affected parts twice a day has also been known to bring relief.

When everything has failed. My humble opinion and advice would be to just leave the damn acne or pimples to nature to sort out! It is a really sobering fact to appreciate that nature sometimes tends to be the best doctor!

24. The Stomach, gateway to you' re a man' s heart?

We all have had stomach problems of varying degrees. As long as we eat, the stomach will always remind us about itself. But first learn the basics. The stomach is a digestive organ, its role is to break down the food we eat, it also a receptor of the drinks we take. It produces stomach juices, hydrochloric acid that help dissolve the food we take. The simplest disturbance of stomach function is dyspepsia. Dyspepsia is a temporary condition by which the stomach warns us when we are doing well to it. It's characterized by simple stomach upsets in the form of short lived vomiting, regurgitations of food, pain in the abdomen. Often, caused by taking more than our stomachs can take, at any particular time, or some taking some irrigative substances. We see this often with children being started on a hard diet from a liquid diet they are used to. Sometimes the stomach just feels full, even when we haven't taken much food. Lose appetite. The stomach is served by along nerve called the Vagus nerve which goes all the way to our brain. This nerve is responsible for sending messages of hunger or satiety to our brains, so that the brain centre can be reminded to stop sending messages to make us want to eat or make us want to look for food. Dyspepsia is not a serious condition; it often passes without any serous treatment or by simple use of milk or use of some basic antacids. The other affliction we can have is cancer of the stomach, not very common in this part of the world. But when it occurs it leads one to have terrible loss of appetite, lose weight, and develop terrible pains and bleedings. Cancer is a dangerous condition when bleeding takes place, it can kill you rather fast. The most frequent condition after dyspepsia is inflammation of the stomach or gastritis, which if s often caused by missing meals, taking some strong drugs, taking alcohol or by developing stress. It comes in form of persistent pains, Loss of appetite and pains, vomiting. It can sometimes be seasonal. Gastritis is a precursor of ulcers if not treated well.

Stomach ulcers are the most serious condition one can get after cancer of the stomach. It's often seasonal. Nowadays scientists understand it as being caused by bacteria. So, stomach ulcers are actually an infective disease, caused by a bacterium called Helico bacter pyrori. But risk factors to having ulcers are like the ones for gastritis i.e. Stress, missing of meals, drugs, alcohol and cigarette smoking. Ulcers produce pains in the stomach 30 minutes after taking food is they are situated in the stomach and 2 hrs. After taking food if they situated lower down in the duodenum or the end of the stomach as it enters the region of your intestines or colon.

Diagnosis

You establish the presence of stomach disorders by:

- A highly suggestive history of abdominal pains on an empty stomach or shortly after taking food.

Special x/rays called barium meals can be done as special investigations.

You can also have a look at the walls of the stomach by some special equipment called gastroscopy.

Treatment

Treatment of ulcers is often accomplished by avoiding irritants like hot spices, alcohol, cigarettes, giving antacids together with antibiotics which may include Amoxicillin and Flagyl, given over a long period.

 A word on the role of stress in the development of gastritis and ulcers... Stress leads to over production of hydrochloric acids in the stomach, so when the stomach is empty this has the propensity of leading it to eat itself! For this reason, milk is often advised as first line defence for stomach upsets, as it calms down the stomach and duodenal walls.

 Surgery is the last resort in the treatment of ulcers and is very useful when the stomach has early cancer lesions. Let us start with "synonyms". Hypertension, High blood BP, High blood, all mean increased high blood pressure, or simply what is in the street is called BP. Not exactly accurate but can do!

25. High blood pressure

First learn the basics. Blood gets pumped from the left side of the heart to the lungs and body through the aorta (the biggest blood vessel in your body) and the Pulmonary artery, about the only arteries which are" wrongly" named as they carry deoxygenated blood to the lungs (all other arteries in the body carry oxygenated blood). All veins should carry deoxygenated blood to the heart.

Blood Pressure is under the regulation of:

1. The heart thrust or power. The more thrust the heart has the more is the blood pressure and the other way around. The size of the heart may increase in muscles!

2. The size and elasticity or the tone of the blood vessels

3. The action of hormones or substances like adrenalin, no-adrenaline, vasopressin, progesterone, thyroxin and others as they influence various organs. Adrenalin for stance has the propensity of constricting the blood vessels, while progesterone may relax them. Adrenalin this was may increase the thrust of the heart, the blood pressure goes up, and the pulse rises. 4. The amount of blood, water, salts in the vessels. Calcium increases the tonus of the blood vessels, tightens them up, in a way. Sodium levels regulates the amount of water in the body by changing the osmolality or "attractiveness" of the contents of blood vessels. This is important to understand as the treatment is aimed at different levels. Everyone has

BP, in the same way we all have temperature! So, you see saying someone has BP is not exactly sensible! What to remember is that high BP is not always a disease; it becomes one when it is persistent. In the same way, low BP which we hear people saying they suffer from is rarely a disease but a condition due to some other disturbance in the body. For this reason, we shall not discuss it here

What Can Cause High BP?

1. Mostly unknown or idiopathic-So called, essential hypertension.

2. As a symptom of some other condition like kidney disease, cancer of the brain, increased levels of fats in the vessels or atherosclerosis

3. Increased levels of stress which leads to increased sustained levels of vascular active substances like adrenalin 4. Diseases of the heart or lungs which may cause increased thrust of the heart. In other words it can be primary where no cause can be pin pointed or secondary where another condition leads to raise in BP. There could be some form genetic disposition to hypertension that means it may run in families.

What Really Happens?

When blood pressure is raised the heart gets to work overtime in order to compensate for the deficit in blood reaching the cells. You tend to have heart palpitations. The brain can suffer from spasms or bleedings called strokes, where small vessels rupture as they are under increased stress. Oxygen does not get to the organs in adequate doses, hence you find the brain getting confused, for example, or the heart failing. Or the kidneys failing, or the lungs being flooded by fluids (pulmonary oedema). Increased BP is particularly dangerous in the pregnant mother, it can lead to strokes, seizures, coma or loss of the baby in utero or womb. But we won't go in detail on this one as it is entirely a different ball game! A single reading of increased blood pressure is not deemed a disease as it can happen after fright, eating, walking upstairs or doing exercises. If this persists beyond the normal of 140/90 mm Hg over a period of time, this is deemed as disease.

Treatment of high BP

 -Vasodilators are used. These drugs widen the size of the vascular system, hence dropping BP -calming drugs as far as stress levels are concerned -Treatment of the original condition if known - use of calcium inhibitor drugs like Nifedipine or better known as Adalat

-Use of diurectics which reduce the levels of water in the vessels, like Moduretic, Diurin, Lasix - Diet control of increased salts and fats -monthly check ups of levels of BP Reduce the risk of having raised BP by: - Reduction of intake of salt and fats - Exercising more - Increase intake of veggies and fruits - Reduce your stress levels Hypertension has no definitive treatment but it can be controlled! Also note that drugs may have their own side effects on the body; Nifedine may produce headaches, Aldomet or Methyldolda may lead to impotency in the male, diuretics like Lasix may dehydrate the body. This is the reason we don't encourage self-treatment of blood pressure!

26. Joint pains

Otherwise known as arthritis. This is the affliction of the joints, their inflammation leading to pain, increased warmth of the joint as well as limitation in their use. Though we often say joint pains mean arthritis, we should understand that not all joint pains are arthritis.

What we often see in the clinic set up are a group of inflammatory bone diseases such as back aches, osteo arthritis, rheumatoid arthritis, gouty arthritis. Common to all is extreme pain! Who has never had back pains? Back pains are as common as is headache in human life.

Pains in the neck and lower back are often as a result of degenerative changes (related to age or pressure) in the spine, the vertebra, as you learnt in your primary school science is a nest of nerves going to the hands and legs. Here in also passes the v major blood vessels to your head. When the spaces between the vertebrae decreases for one reason or the other, this may irritate the various nerves passing out of the spinal cord, these as you know send impulses to your head. Small growths   called osteophytes   may grow out, as a consequence of irritations in the joint. This can cause further pricking on the nerves, resulting in pains. The pains are not only localized in the back but can go all the way to to the legs and arms. Sometimes a person may lose use of arms and legs or get some form of weakness on the muscles of the face (we call this facial palsies or strokes of the face. This denegation or changes may be age related or as I earlier mentioned be as result of extreme pressure on the back due to wrong posture or heavy work. As you know or should know the skeleton is but a support structure for the rest of the body. Sometimes even stress can cause pains in the back and neck. When the spaces become extremely small, operation may be the only option to separate the bones. However sometime simple physio is often helpful or simply avoiding lifting heavy objects or doing work that causes too much pressure of the back. Those with heavy bodies have an increase chance of getting more problems with the back, as the skeletons struggles to support the heavy load!

As far as gouty arthritis is concerned, this is a result of the collection of urea in the joints and urea acts as some form of poison exciting or irritating the nerves, making the joint swell and pain, limiting activity of the concerned joint. Its common knowledge that eating too much red meat may lead to over production of this urea. Sufferers are therefore well advised to reduce or totally avoid taking too much red meat.

27. The Killer under your bed

She kills millions of people a year, she feeds on victims' blood, and she attacks at night and then vanishes in the dawn...
We are not talking of vampires here-We are talking about the mosquitoes...

Did you know as we grapple with Ebola, malaria is wreaking havoc especially among the children?

207 million suffered from malaria in 2012 alone
625 000 died in the same period of one year. Out of this77% were children

1500 children daily die from malaria

And believe me, you can't treat it by chanting prayers and sprinkling oil from Nigerian T.B Joshua

28. Increased weight-The Silent Killer!

Everybody seems to know that increase weight is a problem, to what extent and what to do about it presents difficulties that have in the recent times produced a rolling business in weight reduction programmes and so-called cures. In this page, we shall try to explain what obesity is, how it comes about and what not to do or believe as regards weight control.
First the basics: Normal weight should be presumed to be your height in centimetres minus a hundred. That is if

your height is 175 centimetres, your optimum weight should be around 175-100=75 kg. But note this is only an approximation and not cast in stone, but it's pretty a good one! The more exact measurement if you are the serious type is to take your body mass index (BMI) which is weight in kg(s) divided by the square of your height in metres. This is the formula below:

BMI=Weight/H to the power 2

Example: Your weight is 70 kg, your height is 1.7 metres, which means the square of 1, 7 is 2.89, divide this into your weight of 70, gives an approximate value of 24, so your BMI would be 24.

BMI is a better way to analyse your weight as regards your height.

BMI =Less 15 would be regarded as underweight

Between 15 to 25 would largely be regarded as within normal ranges, and anything above 30-35 as overweight to obese.

Problems related to increased weight:

-Difficulties in breathing as the body struggles to raise the fat tissue in from of the chest and abdomen. Your lungs fail to expand fully. And we all know the less oxygen from the lungs that gets in your body, the worse your general health status would be.

- Obesity may mess up with your hormones, producing disturbed levels which may lead to infertility or difficulties in conceiving.

-Obesity may lead to increased poor function of the fat heart, leading to increase fluid retention in your body, which eventually may lead to increased high blood pressure.

- Increased weight is a risk factor in heart attacks and heart problems as it promotes fat deposition in the coronary arteries, the arteries that service your heart.

- Increased weight may disturb the work of your kidneys as more and more fluids settles in your body, the kidneys can fail, this can also lead to disturbed electrolyte balance in your body , which in turn may disturb the work of several organs in your body...top of which is your heart, brain , and lungs! A vicious cycle is produced which is very difficult to treat.

-Increased weight can lead to poor physical activity in general and in particular to poor sexual performance in both females and men.

In other words increased weight and problems it can cause would demand a text book of its own, but for all practicable purposes, I think I have scared the shit out of you adequately with the above! So perhaps let us talk on what causes it before we can discuss what to do about it.

Causes of increased weight

- Genetic factors-Some people, whatever they do are just born to be fat, although this again can be reduced!

- Over eating

- Poor physical activity. Here you are not burning enough of the fats, the engine oil, you are taking in!

- Intake of high fat containing foods producing high cholesterol levels

- Too much junk food

- Kidney diseases

What can you do about it?

-Throw away the keys to your kitchen and be more active in your life style is the only sure way of controlling your weight. Sounds funny, but it is true. In other words, watch how much and what enters your trap door, the mouth! I have often asked people if they ever have seen a fat prisoner!

This is not to say you need to miss meals, no! Increase in take of fresh veggies and fruits, be more active.

Remember, there are no herbs or drinks (lemon, garlic) nor tablets that can control your weight. Keep away from being cheated by charlatans!

29. Asthma

Learn a little about asthma, also known as bronchial asthma. Hopefully you may help yourself and those being mistreated by some people, being cheated or wrongly treated by some health workers. Or you may help your neighbour or that asthmatic pupil.

What is it? -it's just a chronic inflammatory disorder of the breathing apparatus. Times gone past, we used to think it was an allergic disease, but it is not!

Bronchial Asthma is an inflammatory disease of the air way characterized by repeated difficulties in breathing. Well we all have suffered breathing difficulties from time to time but when this repeat, often wheezy with some irritating cough chances are you have asthma.

What causes it? - Not well understood but heightened

responsiveness of the air way is the root cause accompanied by some inflammation. It can how ever be triggered by...
- animals with fur
-dust
-allergies
-cold
-cockroaches
-physical exercise
-aerosols
-smoke
-pollen
-some drugs such as Reserpine, Aspirin
-strong emotional expressions
symptoms are often as I said accompanied by cough which is worse at night, tight chest, wheezy respirations and this can be seasonal in nature.
The wheeze is a high-pitched sound; usually on breathing out. This is as a result of...
1. Constriction of the airways
2. Swelling or inflammation of the concerned part
3. Mucus production and plugging of the air way

We have heard traditionalists in Zambia and Africa telling you that asthma cannot be handled by health workers, but the truth is though it has no definite treatment health workers can control it. Asthmatic people with "treatment" can continue to lead very productive physical lives or attend school. Treatment here means management!
Fortunately though, some children can grow out of

asthma without any problems.

Diagnosis-we use the suggestive history you give us, often the chest has no changes on x-ray, though some times when someone has had it for too long, and lungs seem hyper inflated. The stethoscope (don't bite your tongue trying to pronounce this one!) may reveal wheezes on listening to the chest, although a quiet chest can point to very serious condition!

In some advanced centres instruments such as spirometers which measure inhaled and out haled air can be used, but they are not often necessary!

What to do when you see someone in an attack.
-turn them on their side, don't put anything in their mouth such as water or other objects, then call a health worker, not try to give any tablets!

For health workers- please stop using Ventolin tablets as maintenance for treatment for Asthmatics, this is currently discouraged as Ventolin has too many side effects (Like speeding up heart rate) Treat the sufferer with an in haler or aerosol, oxygen, and for prevention use long term corticosteroid inhalers like beclomethasone taken twice a day, as puffs. Aminophylline intravenous injection slowly may save life in an emergency or just use a nebulizer to control the patient. You may repeat nebulization's every 15 minutes if the attack is not controlled.

Therefore, we shall say there are things we can give you the sufferer called reliever drugs, and for long term use

controller drugs are used, better given when in aerosol form!
Please asthma can kill, always" treat" it properly! For sufferers avoid triggers mentioned above individually.

30.   Fibroids of the womb

These are growths of the womb or uterus, sometimes called fibromyoma or simply fibroids of the uterus

Causes:

1. Largely unknown

2. Sometimes assumed to be caused by hormonal changes

Types:

1. That which grow on the womb, on top of it, called subseries

2. That which grow inside the muscles of the womb called, intramural fibroids

3. That which grow in the empty space of the womb inside, called sub mucosal 4 rare ones which can be a combination or simply grow on the neck of the womb

Complaints of the woman with fibroids:

Complaints will largely depend on location and size. Can range from abdominal pains, heavy prolonged periods, bleedings in between periods, to persistent foul-smelling discharge; especially when there is secondary infection to the intra-mucosal fibroids. Fibroids can sometimes cause habitual abortions (abortions more than two times). In short it is:

1. Pain abdominal –this is usually related to the tumour pressing of the nearby nerves as it grows.

2. Irregular bleedings from the womb

3. Painful periods Fibroids when left for a long time may lead to cancer of the uterus

How are they diagnosed?

1. Complaints and history

2. By the health worker doing a vaginal examination

3. Ultra- sound scanning

Treatment

Will largely depend on the location and size and sometimes the age of the woman. If the woman is approaching menopause and the symptoms can be tolerated a bit, nothing is done as they often regress spontaneously. Otherwise, the womb may be cleaned with what is called dilation and curettage or " D and C", with a sample of curettings being sent for laboratory investigation to rule out cancer. Most often, fibroids may lead doctors to carry out surgical treatments in form of simple removals or myomectomy, all the way to cutting out the entire womb called hysterectomy. There is no known treatment with tablets, other than pain killers to relieve the pains. Neither can they be treated by prophets as we often hear on some television programmes by overzealous miracle men! No one should die from fibroids. They can be cured (I have yet to see a woman die from fibroids in my entire 30 yr. Gynae practice!) So, don't get cheated!

31.   Flu

Flu is probably the number one affliction of mankind, but its poorly understood and often mishandled. For this reason, let us clear the air. Flu is caused by a virus, not by bacteria and remember in the previous discussion we said viruses are very minute organisms with no life of their own outside host cells, whereas bacteria do live independently of the host. There are probably more than 1000 types of flu viruses that from time to time may attack humans or even some other animals and birds. Surely you have heard of the Asian bird flu that has resulted in deaths of thousands of chickens in Asia, sometimes such avian flu viruses may cross over to infect humans as well. We all know the symptoms of flu, they range from a simple stuffy and running nose, sneezing, sore throat to a dry cough or red eyes, headache. When the virus is at its simplest it only causes what we call coryza or "cold"-sneezing, stuffy nose, sore throat and dry cough but when a rise in temperature is added, and some other symptoms of intoxication like body aches and headaches, then the Coryza becomes a flu. Severe flu often accompanied by loss of appetite and severe body aches and headaches, as well as feelings of tiredness. These symptoms are a result of the body trying to kill off the viruses and releasing toxins as the battle rages between the white blood cells of the body and the viruses. Sometimes flu can kill but it's often non-fatal. Flu can be a major cause of lost time in workers; decreased productivity, through missing work, as people try to recover from it. The thinking that flu is caused by cold weathers is not true. Yes, in cold weather flu epidemics increase, but it's only because in cold weathers people tend to stay indoors in groups, thereby increasing its infectiveness. Flu can be very contagious, just a few drops- lets of cough is all it needs to jump from one human to the other. In colder countries like Ice land and the cold areas of Siberia in Russia where temperatures can drop to below -32 degrees or less, we don't find an increased number of flu cases different from the one in temperate or tropical regions. So cold is not the cause of flu! And you may have sometime seen children or some people who quite comfortably swim in icy waters without developing any flu! You will meet some "flu jabs" on the market, some form of vaccines. The problem is it's often very difficult to pin down all the variants of flu for vaccinations to make any impact. You can have four on the market, for four different types, but then you can get a completely different strain, not covered by the vaccine. Sometimes flu can complicate into some other serious respiratory infections like Pneumonia or affect the muscles of the heart as in Myocarditis. So, when flu prolongs or symptoms are getting worse it is advisable to seek medical opinion. What is important to remember about flu is that it's a viral infection and does not therefore demand use of any antibiotics. You can really not kill viruses by use of antibiotics. Am sure you are all aware of the Amoxicillins, the Penicillin V, and the Erythromycins, the Septrins which people are exposed to, or expose themselves too, unnecessarily. The use of antibiotics in treatment of flu must be strongly discouraged as it is not only costly but encourages resistance of bacteria to them. This is one of the reasons we are currently having super bugs that are becoming increasingly difficult to treat in hospitals or community.

What can you do?

When your child or your self is afflicted by flu use simple remedies as symptomatic measures; Panadols for headaches, body aches and fever, soothing warn drinks like honey or tea for dry throats, some nasal drops for blocked nostrils (for a short period). Cough mixtures so popular with people outside health settings are not necessary! Some people may take vitamin C, but its role in flu has not been proven to be especially more useful than any other vitamin. But it's a harmless thing vitamin to take, anyway (vitamin C may help in absorption of iron in the stomach, may also help in would healing). The flu will take its cause regardless!

32 Broncho Pneumonia

Pneumonia, especially in children, is a major killer; it's only probably second to malaria in the African continent. Pneumonia is a term we use to define the inflammation of the lung

The basics: All the organs in the body get oxygen from the lungs. There are two lungs, one in each part of the chest serviced by two branches of the pulmonary artery from the right side of the heart, which carry deoxygenated blood to them. The right lung has three lobes while the left has two lobes or main parts. Hence you will hear of lobular pneumonia being mentioned sometimes, which just means the inflammation or affliction of part of the lung with distinct borders. When the inflammation is spread over more lobes, it's called simply bronco pneumonia. Two veins from each side of the lungs run to the left upper part of the heart, the atrium. What more, they are called veins but they carry oxygenated blood when all the veins in the body carry deoxygenated blood. The pulmonary arteries carry deoxygenated blood from the heart! This is the only place you find arteries and veins roles reversed!

What causes pneumonia?

Pneumonia is caused mainly by bacteria, although viruses and fungus are also known to cause the disorder to a lesser extent. Among the commonest causers of pneumonia are bacteria, common is, haemophilus influenza, streptococcus, staphylococcus, pneumococcus. The causative bug enters the lungs through in haled air or may be carried via blood from some other site in the body. Some conditions can lead to what is called secondary pneumonia, a form of complication, such as measles, influenza, bronchitis and even heart failure associated with what is called as static Pneumonia, mostly due to immobility. Pneumonia can also be caused by inhalation of toxic fumes or burns but we won't discuss this here, as it is a rather a rare cause for the pathology.

Symptoms: The patient complains of excessive weakness, headache, persistent cough which can be dry or with sputum, the body temperature rises to 38 -39 degrees centigrade, the breathing becomes rather laboured and fast (normal respiratory rate in adults is between 16-20), the pulse rate rises to above normal. (The normal ranges from 60-80 beats per minute), loss of appetite is observed and in very small children inability to breast feed. Parents must note that any small child or baby with a fever, refusal to feed, fast breathing or laboured breathing signifies always Broncho pneumonia and not flu! If such a child is not quickly attended to can easily die! Diagnosis is based on history of persistent cough accompanied by fever. As I said before, any fast breathing, or laboured breathing in a small child always suggests pneumonia! The full blood count reveals a rise in white cells which normally range between 4000-6 000 per ml. This is because the infection leads to mobilization of the white cells in the defence system to fight the infection. The x ray shows thickening of the lung tissue. However, X-ray is not imperative in management of children as the signs are rather very obvious. We have seen cases where treatment is delayed because an x ray has not been done- this is dangerous and bad medical practice; it's incorrect! Treatment where possible it's often better to use intravenous antibiotics, Oxygen is given to the affected patient through the nose.

Prevention Adequate balanced diet, non-smoking, less use of alcohol and in children avoidance of flues or other viral infections like measles and exposure to cold is important. I should add that in Zambian hospitals and other African countries many children die of pneumonia because mothers take their children late for treatment. A lot of time is spent on things that do not work like cough mixtures or oral short-lived antibiotics. This is one dangerous disease and parents are well advised to seek medical help fast!

33. Persistent Mouth Odours

Does your mouth give off a persistent smell from it? Do you perhaps know someone having such?

This condition is sometimes called halitosis and it's a cause for many stressful times in some people, more so, that the recognition of the cause or even treatment appears to some, not to be so simple. When I speak of mouth odours am referring to persistent mouth odours.

The mouth can smell from the following:

1. Type of food- You know very well the persistent smell that comes from a mouth of a garlic lover. Garlic as you will find out is not easily removed by simply cleaning the teeth. 2. Caries teeth-When the teeth have some holes in them, food particles are bound to fall in them, disintegrate, rot and may give off a smell. Teeth brushes do not reach the depth of these holes in the teeth so cleaning the mouth may not bring relieve. 3. Gum diseases, diseases of the tonsils-Any suppurative (pus giving) condition occurring in the mouth can lead to mouth odours. Rarely, lung conditions such as lung abscess can give off odours, but the truth is they such are rarely missed! 4. The diseases of the stomach-This condition is hardly suspected in many sufferers, but it's the main cause of difficult to diagnose persistent mouth

odours. The thing is the sufferer develops some form of "internal" allergy to proteins. Food ingested tends to produce high levels of substances skatol, indols which give off very strong smells through the mouth. One needs to approach one's health worker to rule out stomach disease in every case of persistent mouth odours not due to the top three mentioned. Treatment may take weeks, apart from avoiding such foods which may be found to be promoting the condition talking about mouth hygiene, what we should perhaps mention here is that it is senseless to clean your teeth in the morning! The food we take carries with it many substances and bacteria, it's advisable therefore to clean teeth after each meal. Or at least, before settling down to sleep. Cleaning teeth in the morning prevalent among many of us is really doing some ting after the bacteria in our mouths have had a whole night preying on our teeth! I know this sounds weird

But that is the truth; teeth are better cleaned before settling to bed! Any honest dentist out there will tell you the same thing! It does not make much sense to clean and then deposit a new baggage of germs with our foods with our breakfast!

34. General health tips

You got to remember these. Use them in your daily life, spread them around to your loved ones, to your friends, so that they too may be empowered, for as they say, knowledge is indeed power!

1. Cough Mixtures-Do not try to stop harmless dry cough on yourself or your child. Cough is but a defence mechanism by the body, do not suppress it. Avoid use of cough mixtures, they a have no role in modern medical practice.

2. Do not take antibiotics indiscriminately without a proper diagnosis from a health worker. Always ask the health worker who gives antibiotics what indeed is wrong with you. Indiscriminate of use of antibiotics is harmful to everyone as it promotes resistance and is often a waste of money.

3. Do not take drugs for short lived diarrhoea or abdominal pains or back aches, or even headaches, these often subside independently.

4. Do not take antibiotics for flu. Flu is caused by viruses, you cannot kill viruses by use of antibiotics.

5. Look for stomach problems if you have a persistent mouth odour after ruling out problems in the mouth!

6. Every woman should get a pap smear at least once in two yrs., a man after 40 years of age have his prostate checked through a simple blood test called PSA

7. There is no drug that can drop your weight. Weight control is a matter of controlling what is going in your mouth, how much, increased veggies and fruits, active mode of life, is the only sure way to go.

8. Coca Cola and Cafenol can never prevent pregnancy after unprotected sex. 9. Fever is not a disease but a symptom of a disease

10. Lumber puncture does not kill the patient, what kills is the meningitis that the patient may be having.

12. There is no drug or herb that can enlarge your organs

13. Tea, lemon juice cannot be used to drop your weight

14. When you are asleep, you really do not know that you are asleep

15. Dreams predict the past, they never predict the future

16. Marijuana never killed a man, but alcohol does!

17. Contrary to popular belief, your heart is not the seat of love; it's the seat of your blood. Your brain is where our love sits

18. Brain cells once dead do not regenerate!

19. Mostly, impotence is a psychological condition, never physical

20. Stress or worry can make a woman miss her periods without being pregnant. 21. A man's chest contains as many ribs as a woman's

22. This we mentioned under sugar disease, but it does not harm to repeat, as repletion is the mother of learning, they say. Taking more Sugar does not cause diabetes but may make its control more difficult.

35. Infertility -The basics…

Also known as bareness by my mother and yours. We define barrenness or infertility as the inability of a couple to sheer off springs. This inability becomes infertility when the couple has had unprotected regular sex for a period of one year.
Let me repeat this point, you got to stay, having tried for a whole period of one year, not six months or even 9 months! Regular sex must be understood as at least two or thrice in a week. Note, not number of times but days in a week.

We further differentiate primary infertility as when couple has had no child ever and secondary infertility when after a child or two the couple does not conceive any more children for a period equal to one year, having not been using any contraceptives or prevention what so ever. It can be further affect only the male, female or both partners. In fact the cause of infertility is found to be related to the female partner in 50 % of cases, male partners about 40% and both partners may have problems at 10%.Therefore the way sometimes men in Zambia, and Africa as whole want to blame the female as the cause is born out of ignorance!

Causes of infertility:

in females-Blocked tubes at almost 90% of the cases

- Hormonal disturbances

-obesity-which invariably lead to hormonal disturbance

- Growths in the womb, like fibroids which may lead to disturbed implantation of the fertilized egg and further growth of the embryo

- Stress, which acts on higher centres of the brain disturbing the normal cycle of releases of hormonal precursors

- Sometimes no cause is found!

Male infertility- Reduced sperm count, the normal being about 50-250 million per ml of sperm

-Absent sperms or azoospermia, either in -born or acquired.

- Surgery on the Vas deferens, the tube that caries the sperms, leading to kinking or narrowing

- urethral strictures

- Unknown

Investigations and diagnosis

For the male a sperm count is all that is required. Normal Spermogram has active sperms, normal ones, not with double heads, has good motility, and does not contain pus cells, sperms about 50 -250 million per ml of semen (the normal ejaculate is close to 2mls!). An Urologist can then be called upon to make further evaluation when the sperm count is low or absent.

For the female after the normal blood and urine tests for both partners, we advise hormonal tests. Ultrasound to see the nature of the ovaries, a special x-ray called Hystero-Salpingography (HSG) is a must

Sometimes x-rays of the pituitary gland in the head, the organ from which the hormones come from may be necessary.

Treatment is often done according to findings of the cause, but believe me does not involve prophet's help, as many Zambians seem to think!

Avoid undue stress and worry for both partners, avoid for the male working in areas with extreme temperatures, extreme tiredness and too frequent sexual activity, avoid intake of too much alcohol and avoid smoking.

Where everything fails the couple can adopt or go for expensive in vitro (or in viva) fertilization in advanced medical centres.

36. What we were not taught about drugs!

1. Yes you guessed right, alcohol is a drug and a common one at that! Taking one drink at a party and becoming a constant heavy drinker who loses control of himself frequently are two different things altogether. People who drink every day sooner find themselves more and more dependent on alcohol or at least they start thinking they need a drink every day. They begin to drink more and more and soon lose control of their faculties; they can no longer control their drinking. The situation gets worse even though the person understands that they are truly harming themselves. Neither people who cannot control the way they drink nor the amount are called alcoholics. Alcoholism is an illness that becomes worse with each bout of drink. The sad thing is teenage alcoholics are increasing at a very fast pace.

No one can quarrel that drinking makes a person's mind to work more slowly, their speech is slurred, muscles and reaction time gets impaired. The inhibitory role of the brain in each one of us is eroded leading to violent behaviours, lose behaviours, risky behaviours. More so the alcoholic may sooner lose his job or fail to cater for his family and many are in denial!

Alcohol endangers automobile drivers leading to terrible accidents, often involving innocent lives. Since your brain centre is numbed, you may react violently in what is really a normal situation. Finally, alcohol damages the brain cells and be reminded that unlike skin cells they never regenerate, once gone they are gone! Your liver may get damaged, kidneys and many other organs follow suit. Cirrhosis of the liver often caused by alcohol is not advisable, and it results in only one thing-death! Sometimes I think the modern man will really laugh at us for using alcohol so much, at weddings and parties!

2. Smoking- Though many of us do smoke cigarettes, none of us can defend this bad habit! We all know, or should know smoking not only can cause cancer but can damage your organs, all organs as cigarette nicotine is really a habit-forming drug. Besides the tar contained in cigarettes has its own effect on all organs. Why then do we humans smoke? I wish I could answer this one, often we associate stress, boredom as the cause but this when deeply considered is just not true, scientifically. Smoking is just a bad habit and habits die very hard!

3. Glue- When sniffed this makes you feel drunk and dizzy. It can damage your blood cells and your liver. One word from me avoid glue, it's nothing to do with sticking stuff up! Strange we use similar words for two different things…. humans!!

4. Sleeping pills- This may include the common Valium and Phenobarbitals, which we commonly meet in hospital use. In bad hands, they can damage your liver and mess up your memory and brain cells big time. They inhibit the brain centres and are habit forming. One word from me, if it isn't given by a health worker avoid it!

5. Cough Mixtures-They contain codeine, a chemical which is made from opium. Codeine is habit forming. Now

you understand why we are no longer providing you with cough mixtures in hospitals, but unfortunately many of them are really popular across the counter drugs. The private pharmacies and medical practitioners who should know better are particularly notorious at dishing out bottles of cough mixtures. In fact, let me digress a bit and emphasize that suppressing a defence mechanism that is cough is no longer medically sensible, but common sense is not so common after all! And really science does change, keep up with the latest views!

6. Marijuana-I think you have been waiting to hear what I say on this one, for there is so much miss- information regarding marijuana out there. This is a plant widely grown in many African countries, South America and Afghanistan (Zambia, included!).It rarely needs any serious tendering when growing. You had better listen to Sinkamba, he has a point!
The smoker feels light headedness and may lose his sense of judgment, he may do things that are out of character for him. Marijuana now un- banned in a horde of states in US and Denmark has very useful medicinal uses, apart from bringing in huge sums of money to sellers. We use marijuana among other things in pain control and in the treatment of nausea for people on chemo therapy for cancer. The hullabaloo we hear about its dangers is perhaps exaggerated and misplaced. It is not such a strong drug in habit forming arsenal. Surely none has died ever using marijuana as compared to alcohol! My verdict-time to change our attitudes to this very useful drug, it's

not only a money earner for any struggling economy but has beneficial medical effects.

7. Heroin-This is a strong drug and some people erroneously think it is marijuana! When this drug is injected into the skin or veins it brings about such stronger need for more that the addict does not care what he does to get it, can kill or steal! The user from a high feeling increasingly becomes weak. Heroin is so addictive that users often resort to ever increasing doses to get high; it may cause premature death, as you certainly remember how many singers have succumbed to it, some of them really big stars

8. LCD –Powerful man made chemical whose correct name if you can allow me is lysergic acid diethylamide. Its users often end up with bizarre mental reactions and may lead to distorted sense of touch, smell or feeling; hearing may be distorted as well. It may cause not only raised blood pressure but can totally mess up one's appetite, causes paranoia and is been often implicated in accidental deaths as the heart gets affected

37. Persistent Mouth Odours revisited

Does your mouth give off a persistent smell from it? Do
you perhaps know someone having such?
This condition is sometimes called halitosis and it's a
cause for many stressful times in some people, more so
that the recognition of the cause or even treatment
seems, to many, not to be so simple. When I speak of
mouth odours am referring to persistent mouth odours.
The mouth can smell from the following:
1. Type of food- You know very well the persistent smell
that comes from a mouth of a garlic lover. Garlic as you
will find out is not easily removed by simply cleaning the
teeth.
2. Caries teeth-When the teeth has some holes in them,
food particles are bound to fall in them, disintegrate, rot
and may give off a smell. Teeth brushes do not reach the
depth of these holes in the teeth so cleaning the mouth
may not bring relieve.
3. Gum diseases, diseases of the tonsils-Any suppurative
(pus giving) condition occurring in the mouth can lead to
mouth odours. Rarely lung conditions such as lung abscess
can give off odours, but the truth is they such are rarely
missed!
4. The diseases of the stomach-This condition is hardly
suspected in many sufferers, but it's the main cause of
difficult to diagnose persistent mouth odours. The thing is
the sufferer develops some form of "internal" allergy to
proteins. Food ingested tends to produce high levels of

substances skatol, indols which give off very strong smells through the mouth. One needs to approach one's health worker to rule out stomach disease in every case of persistent mouth odours not due to the top three mentioned. Treatment may take weeks, apart from avoiding such foods which may be found to be promoting the condition

talking about mouth hygiene, what we should perhaps mention here is that it is senseless to clean your teeth in the morning! The food we take carries with it many substances and bacteria; it's advisable therefore to clean teeth after each meal. Or at least, before you settle down to sleep. Cleaning teeth in the morning prevalent among many of us is really doing something after the bacteria in our mouths have had a whole night preying on our teeth, after the bacteria have had a field day in out moths! I know this sounds weird but that is the truth, teeth are better cleaned before settling to bed! Any honest dentist out there will tell you the same thing! It does not make much sense to clean and then deposit a new baggage of germs with our foods with our breakfast!

38. Not for under 18's!

Snippet of sexual problems
First things first. Let us look at male sexual response.
1. Desire- This is just a subjective feeling for wanting to copulate, or let us call it, thinking following sight of your "animal" for slaughter!!
2. Arousal-The wish for copulation leads to a state of heightened excitement leading to erection of the male organ in response to physical stimulus or further thoughts.
3. Erection -Sustained rush of blood to the male organ, increase in size and length
4. Ejaculation and orgasm-The male organ discharges its arsenal, leading to heightened feeling of satisfaction, jerking of muscles, rapid heartbeats and respirations, sweating
5. Luminescence- The organ returns to its rest status, loss of erection

6. Refractory phase -During this period no erection is possible despite stimulation, may take 25 minutes or less in younger people and even up to a week in those above 50 yrs. of age.

For the female, we may see similar reactions with nipples, and clitoris taking on erect positions, an increase of wetness in the vagina. Orgasm is the same like in males and a period of luminescence may be accompanied by increased wish to sleep. But the female being a passive participant in the act is often capable of engaging in continuous sexual activity.

Most common sexual disorder is the failure of the male to have an erection. This can be due to medical conditions like diabetes, hypertension, side effects of drugs like Aldomet and others, stress, tiredness, extreme fears, fears to satisfy the partner, atherosclerosis or disease of the vascular system. Failure to erect is often due to psychological reasons which may be made worse by the partners being less sensitive with words or the like. So-called erectile dysfunction. -rarely due to physical causes. The other problem the male may face is premature ejaculation, which you may understand to mean the male ejaculates immediately upon penetration or shortly thereafter. This condition is mostly caused by fears of ability to perform. We advise the partner to reduce the rhythmic movements or further stimulation, pinch the male organ with your nails which may lead to a reflex cooling down in the male. Avoid taking alcohol in large quantities. The thing with alcohol is it gives desire and takes away the performance, so to say, with the passage of time.

Frigidity or failure to have orgasm in females is often due to poor technique from the male partner, fear of disease, fear of getting pregnant , stress and sometimes may be in born, but this is very rare .

Most sexual problems can be resolved by un- rushed understanding by both partners, by avoiding use of careless remarks of inadequacy of partner, avoiding of stress and counselling by health personnel if persistent. Males are warned to avoid self-prescription with drugs such as Viagra which could be a danger to their health! The thing to remember is that, sexual feelings do drop with age so do not worry yourself too much!

39. Broncho Pneumonia

Pneumonia especially in children is a major killer; it's only probably second to malaria in the African continent. Pneumonia is a term we use to define the inflammation of the lung

The basics:
All the organs in the body get oxygen from the lungs. There are two lungs, one in each part of the chest serviced by two branches of the pulmonary artery from the right side of the heart, which carry deoxygenated blood to them. The right lung has three lobes while the left has two lobes or main parts. Hence you will hear of lobular pneumonia being mentioned sometimes, which just means the inflammation or affliction of part of the lung with distinct borders. When the inflammation is spread over more lobes, it's called simply bronco pneumonia. Two veins from each side of the lungs run to the left upper part of the heart, the atrium. What more, they are called veins but they carry oxygenated blood when all the veins in the body carry deoxygenated blood. The pulmonary arteries carry deoxygenated blood from the heart! This is the only place you find arteries and veins roles reversed!

What causes pneumonia?
Pneumonia is caused mainly by bacteria, although viruses and fungus are also known to cause the disorder to a lesser extent. Among the commonest causers of pneumonia are bacteria, common is, haemophilus influenza, streptococcus, staphylococcus, pneumococcus. The causative bug enters the lungs through in haled air or may be carried via blood from some other site in the body. Some conditions can lead to what is called secondary pneumonia, a form of complication, such as measles, influenza, bronchitis and even heart failure associated with what is called static Pneumonia, mostly due to immobility. Pneumonia can also be caused by inhalation of toxic fumes or burns but we won't discuss this here, as it is a rather a rare cause for the pathology.

Symptoms:
The patient complains of excessive weakness, headache, persistent cough which can be dry or with sputum, the body temperature rises to 38 -39 degrees centigrade, the breathing becomes rather laboured and fast (normal respiratory rate in adults is between 16-20), the pulse rate rises to above normal. (The normal is 60-80 beats per minute), loss of appetite is observed and in very small children inability to breast feed. Parents must note that any small child or baby with a fever, refusal to feed, fast breathing or laboured breathing signifies always Broncho pneumonia and not flu! If such a child is not quickly attended to can easily die!
Diagnosis
is based on history of persistent cough accompanied by fever.

As I said before, any fast breathing, or laboured breathing in a small child always suggests pneumonia!
The full blood count reveals a rise in white cells which normally range between 4000-6 000 per ml. This is because the infection leads to mobilization of the white cells in the defence system to fight the infection.
The x ray shows thickening of the lung tissue. However, X-ray is not imperative in management of children as the signs are rather very obvious. We have seen cases where treatment is delayed because an x ray has not been done- this is dangerous and bad medical practice; it's incorrect!
Treatment

Where possible it's often better to use intravenous antibiotics, Oxygen is given to the affected patient through the nose.
Prevention
Adequate balanced diet, non-smoking, less use of alcohol and in children avoidance of flues or other viral infections like measles and exposure to cold is important.
I should add that in Zambian hospitals and other African countries many children die of pneumonia because mothers take their children late for treatment. A lot of time is spent on things that do not work like cough mixtures or oral short-lived antibiotics. This is one dangerous disease and parents are well advised to seek medical help fast!

40. Sexually Transmitted Infections

sometimes called STD's referring to diseases which is not exactly saying the same thing. More like HIV infection is not necessarily AIDs. But we can use them interchangeably all the same so long we don't assume too much. Here I will not discuss HIV infection, even though its sexually transmitted infection, but it is a broad topic requiring its own standalone attention, to do justice to it. I will also not discuss the buboes (swellings) as they are not so frequent pathologies in out set up.

I know of no infection that is so unfairly treated as sexually transmitted infections. Sex here seems to be the key but this removes the idea that you can get them through non sexual means as well, as in warts, which you can get by direct contact with the lesions, or by being born with same...Any way controversies aside they are mostly sexually transmitted.

We may divide them into three main groups, those that cause discharges, and those that cause ulcers, and then those that give off growths as in warts.

A) Discharge causing; in both males and females...

1.Gonorrhea- causes by Neisseria Gonococcus germ

2.Chlamydia-caused by Chlamydia Trachomatis bacteria

3. Candidiasis- caused by Candida Albicans, some form of mush room, so to say.

4. Trichomoniasis-caused by Trichomonas bacteria

B) Ulcer causing

1.Chancroid-caused by Chlamydia Trachomatis

2 Syphilis- caused by a germ Treponema Pallidum

3. Herpes simplex lesions- caused by HPV Simplex, a virus

C) Growths like warts caused by Human Papilloma virus, same virus which causes cervical cancer in women

It's not necessary to differentiate the type of discharge as caused by different organisms in the current syndromic approach being used nowadays. Neither is it important to differentiate the character of ulcers. This is so because treatment is taken as nonspecific involving a barrage of injections and tablets. Special mention should be made of warts however which often require cautery or burning by surgical means or very active substances. Often do recur after treatment. As for herpes genitalis- it's a viral eruption needing sometimes only avoidance of sexual activity, however some anti-viral cream (Acyclovir) is sometimes used. Mostly they resolve without any problems. They are often painful small pimples on the private parts.

Long term effects of STIs are blockage of tubes in females causing infertility, narrowing of urethras in males making passing of urine difficult or they may affect the unborn child or even pregnancy as when premature labour is triggered. Or sometimes infections may spread into the abdomen causing pelvic inflammatory diseases in women, swelling of the scrotum in men.

Late syphilis can affect all internal, organs, even the skin, all the way to affecting the brain, where a person may sometimes even become mad.

For this reason STI's must be treated with respect!

41. The Small Guys, own this Earth!

Am not talking about you and me; we are big! Am talking about the really small guys out there, the microbes! First they are the most numerous in the universe. Take your hand and look at it, looks clean? But there are billions shamming and swimming, even after you have killed a few millions by washing your hands in soap. You can really not get rid of them completely. Yes, you may reduce their numbers, but only by an insignificant level. If you want to look at your washed hand with a microscope, you will get shocked at the animals moving, you are bound to see. Likewise, someone rightly once pointed out that your mouth is actually dirtier that your anus! Your mouth gets so many small organisms both living and dead that you would wonder why you are still alive! It's a sobering fact that the food we take in is actually not sterile, it can never be. In fact, if it was we would as people even get sicker!

There are bacteria on your skin in billions, in your colon, in your stomach even in your eyes. There are all over! The only good thing is that about 1 in 1000 are actually harmful organisms, the rest are actually beneficial! These bacteria help in the digestion of our foods and in fighting other harmful cousins in our bodies. They may be number two killer things after HIV and accidents in our time, but we really need them for our survival. The difference between bacteria if you may know and viruses is that while bacteria are assumed to be living things, viruses are not. Viruses are not only much smaller but outside the host cell are useless, they are as good as dead. Give them a host cell and they can wreak havoc, what we have seen with viruses as for yellow fever, Ebola, Zika, HIV among others, or even the well-known flu viruses.

A few years ago the world learnt of the adaptability of some of these organisms when faced with very strange conditions. An un manned Apollo craft which landed on the moon way back in 1967, left a camera behind on the moon, a place which you know has no food nutrients, no air, it's a vacuum, so to say. On being retrieved after two yrs. by the crew of Apollo 12, the camera revealed living organisms upon return to earth! Apparently, this was not a sign of life on the moon but that the bugs had been deposited on the camera when the astronaut was installing it, two yrs. previously, on the moon! However, the germs had lived through a period of no air, water, nor food, with temperatures going as long as -250 degrees centigrade. Now you see, if these small fellows can live in such conditions, you cannot wonder why your soap does nothing to them really! Some of these bugs can survive anything-nuclear reactors, Antarctica, hot springs- anything! Yes, humans may have a developed consciousness but not even that can make them survive in a nuclear reactor or a hot spring!

They are pretty clever chaps at evading death! Take your vomiting, diarrhoea, sneezing, did you know that's the way they get to leave one organism to the next (human beings included). The ones like malaria parasites are even clever, they get into your blood stream before your immune systems can figure them out. In fact, you should know that we feel bad when these organisms multiply in our bodies, not because of what they are doing to our bodies but what our bodies are doing to them! Sickness from an infective agent is due to the fight the body tries to put up against invaders, other than what the invaders themselves are doing. When our white cells kill off bacteria, a lot of substances are produced which are in turn very toxic to our bodies? That's why you find chaps like the flu virus and HIV try to disguise themselves before they end up being killed by our defence white cells. Only a stupid bug kills off its host when it's all dependent on it; only a stupid bug kills off its host quickly. Most are not, because they too may die in the process! This we see with HIV virus which tries to keep the host upon which it is dependent for many years alive, in order that it may continue to reproduce. Ebola virus out breaks is short lived precisely because Ebola kills off its hosts rather too quickly. The flu virus is clever one, when the host gets sicker it quickly jumps to the next, that's why definitive treatment of it is so difficult! The thing about viruses is once they enter the host cells they try to incorporate the hosts DNA or genetic material into their own in order to replicate and survive. For this reason, the host body defence mechanism finds it rather very difficult to attack them, even though they are able to pick out the signs of some foreign invasion. The malaria germ is not so foolish either, it has found a way to run off into an intermediary the mosquito before the client dies!

Next time you claim supremacy on earth among living and dead things think of who really owns this earth! Certainly not humans!

42.   Headaches...

Who hasn't had one?

1. Headache is the only problem i can with conviction tell you that you are not generous with truth if you deny you have never had it

2. Headache is not a disease but a sign or symptom of a problem

3. Did know that most headaches are lifestyle related?

4 Doctors carry a tremendous baggage of info and don't ask them about headaches because they are number one sufferers at this, probably related to worrying about their patients than themselves! Then follows a close second business executives (and you know why!)...then house wives (it's one stressful job, you know!).Remember to thank your mum, for she rarely made you aware of her headaches!

Sales men, for again obvious, reasons are prone to headaches at number four, followed by clerks, farmers (especially during droughts!}

....And you guessed right, manual workers suffer from headaches the least!!

5 Okay a lot of things can cause headaches, close to more than 1000 causes, but some are pretty straight forward like when you have malaria or any infection, a tumour or growth in your head, hypertension or any other chronic disease, or your eyes are straining due to poor eye sight...doctors know all that and that's why they have more headaches than you and me!

6.All headaches can practically be traced to either dilated blood vessels in the head or muscle tension in the head and neck...so therefore, fortunately most headaches, it can be said , have no physical cause one can place their hands on.

7. Migraine....Am sure you all have heard of this one. Migraine headaches though terrible can actually be traced to some form of response to a social or occupational difficulty...the muscles of the neck tense, spreading to the face and focusing on one eye. I won't bore you with the physiology. Save to say that this tension of sustained contractions of the scalp and neck muscles leads to changes on the behaviour of three distinct blood vessels in the head. ....constriction or narrowing-this leads to an aurora, some funny feelings like numbness, tingling sensation, seeing stars, and blind spots, then comes dilation or enlargement which results in pounding pain, nausea, shivering, and finally the last change is sip of fluids into these vessels walls, the vessel walls become hard and literally like pipes, leading to a constant sustainable pain that may last anything from a few hours to a days.

You have heard migraine sufferers shouting that, they feel like dying, but I can tell you, no one really dies out of them, neither do they commit suicide because sooner or later they are back to normal and they know it!!

Migraine and foods---Keep away from triggers that we know can start an attack, like eating chocolates and cheese. Scientists think that it is the chemical Tyramine which is contained in these products that is responsible. But I can attest to cases of migraine being induced by cigarettes and alcohol consumption, even some times coffee and tea...Now shall you stop taking these? Yes, if you are a sufferer and has noticed that these triggers your attacks.... look, it's like asthma, if dust triggers your attacks, you keep away. You are your own physician, I dare say! Let us call it cerebral allergy in cases of migraine, it's all the same...anything can be a trigger!

Stress the number one condition on earth cannot be discounted! So, keep away from stressful situations. Of course, in this computer age with Lusaka or any other cities and towns full of cars with" crazy" drivers it's easier said than done, i should admit.

SELF HELP- migraine sufferers or other headaches can sometimes just help themselves by gentle rotation of their necks and gentle message of the neck of the neck, often this digital pressure on the vessels, the ones i dint want to mention, the temporal arteries, starve the surface supply of blood to the rest of the head and improves the headache. Or take Panadol or aspirin if persists.

Drugs---At times, migraine, if it gets notorious forces the good doctors to prescribe strong drugs like ergotamine tartrate that is often taken below the tongue to relieve the migraine. The only back draw to drug use is you get to use increasing doses and may become addicted. And we know what addiction does, you literally become a moving pharmacy, would you like that?

Relax---Many headaches don't need any treatment, take it easy. Have enough sleep and as we always preach always use correct posture when sitting at work or study, walk

more, don't drive to your toilet! Have some exercises, it often improves blood circulation!!
So next time you have headache, think... are you not the headache

43. The truth about Science!

Don't cheat yourself, we all use science all of us, even those who pour scorn on it. You use science when you use the lift, the toilet, when you boil your tea!
Boiling something is no more that speeding up molecules to collide more quickly to produce heat!
Why do you think high mountain tops like Everest and Kilimanjaro are colder that lower areas when if you use common sense, the higher you go to the sun the hotter it should become?
It's simple really to understand, if you apply your scientific mind to it. The sun is about 93 000 000 miles from earth, so you're going up the mountain has not really gotten you far enough to make any discernible difference. See what I mean? Science is beautiful, science explores, science questions. Nothing is sacred in science, not even your religious beliefs!
Back to the mountain riddle; when you go higher up, the pressure acting on you and the air around you become less and less, therefore the air molecules become distant from each other, the collisions between them becomes rarer, hence less heat is produced. See how nice science makes you unravel seemingly confusing things?
Science's aim is not to disprove the existence of God, but

to make you relate easily to your environment, to understand it better, if that leads you to God or away from Him, it's only accidental, really.

Now, you have heard the fanatics deny that evolution makes sense, yet everyone knows and appreciates black Americans have evolved to have longer hair over time because of where they are. The Norwegians are whiter than the Manchester guys, chicken eggs in Russia, because of snow, are white instead of brown! The black man is black because of the raging sun acting more forcibly on his skin! I hope you won't ask why the monkey does not evolve into you, for evolution takes millions, if not billions of years, and every species have over time evolved separate routes!

Embrace science, move on, and learn! Meaning when you die you don't resurrect, no one ever did, forget the stories! Not until we have sorted out the cryo -science where we shall be able to revive dead bodies after hundreds of years of freezing! Is this so difficult to appreciate? Already we are able to freeze human embryos for ages and revive them to life! Yes, we haven't yet cracked how to make life, but one day, just one day, science will get there! Science is progressive, science never sleeps!

That is of course, if Putin and Donald Trump do not blow us all up into ashes! One day, the unknown will be known, mark my words!

44. Getting things into perspective!

You may have heard the following medical insights that you should not sleep on your right side of your body because
1. Sleeping on the right may lead to oesophageal reflux as the oesophagus or food pipe enters the stomach from the right top; making acid easier to climb up your throat, makes digestion of food much more difficult, and may cause pain along the throat.
2. The heart works better pumping blood to the rest of the body as the aorta, the largest blood vessel, bends to the left as it leaves the heart.
3. The main body of the stomach lies more on the left side, lying on the right side may push the stomach against the pancreatic duct from the pancreas, which makes it difficult for the flow of the pancreatic juice (for digestion of food)
..And other medical hacks

But the truth is neither is sleeping mouth up good for a long time as the tongue may fall behind the throat obstructing your breathing. But also sleeping on the left may impede lymph circulation as the main lymph vessels pass on the left. The spleen lies on the left as well, pressure on it may impede its work of blood cell regulation. The lymphatic system is like a cleaner or drainage system in your body
don't worry, the body is a clever machine and unless you are comatose or too drunk, change of position happens in the night automatically without you even being aware of it. But remember prolonged use of one side may lead to

bed sores and body aches-especially in those who are unconscious. The rule is to change position every two hours at least.

45. The cold season is here!

Let us recap how to navigate thru it, at least medically speaking!
1. Don't take cough mixtures for every cough, take warm fluids, soothing throat things like warm honey. Let cough run its course, it is there to defend you(it's a defence mechanism employed by your body against irritants)
2.But a cough more than two weeks may need medical attention, to rule out some serious infection, especially if it comes with fever or bloody sputum, or it is a wet cough.
3.A small child need to be kept warm all the time, any refusal of feeds, with or without fever, any lethargy, may indicate serious disease and needs a dr to see.
4 Avoid buying antibiotics and using them without prescription from a dr. and also suspect malpractice when the same is given to you by any health worker for simple (uncomplicated) flu.
5 Don't get excited by flu jabs...you are unlikely to protect yourself from catching flu, as the flu jabs cannot cover all possible (viral) causes of flu
4.Pneumonia is a serious ailment, especially in children, and may require admission to a health facility. But not every cough is pneumonia! It could be viral, fungal or

bacterial or even chemical as in inhalation of toxic fumes
...fever is always present in most cases of pneumonia.

5 Not every sore throat requires medications, mostly are
viral, soothe the throat, avoid cold drinks and wait for
nature to sort you out!
6 Above all remember common cold, flu are viral
infections, please do not use anti

46. Stroke._

We can understand stroke to mean failure of function of a
given part of the body, or sometimes even functioning at
a lesser optimal level.
Strokes in the body are caused by disturbed blood and
nerve function in a given organ. Following this we may
divide strokes into'' insults'' or bleeds ,as result of
blockage of passage of blood to a given portion of the
brain or the ischaemic(pronounced ''*iskemik*'') type when
such reduction is due to disruption of adequate blood
supply through for example mere spasm or constriction of
the conduit.
You may recall that the right brain controls the left and
the left controls the right, so when you see weakness on
the right side body, the problem could be in the left brain
and vice versa. This helps doctors to localize the area of
damage in your brain or spine, as it were. You therefore
hear of hemi (from the Latin word meaning half) paresis
or weakness and paralysis (total failure) which means half
of your body is afflicted and quadri-paresis (quadri, the
Latin word for four) or paralysis when all four limbs, the

arms and legs are involved. A growth or tumour in the spine of one's neck would result to loss or reduction of function of the arms and legs and all that which comes below the level concerned. The idea of distinguishing which place is affected involves tapping, pricking different sites on your body by the doctor specialized in nerves or neurologist. However, each doctor has a pretty good idea of basic neurology that is taught in medical school and gathered through experiences as one continues to work. In short then the causes of strokes can be numerous but the main ones are:

1. Nerve damage
2. Infection in the brain disrupting its function, as in HIV/AIDS or Meningitis. We have seen that facial paralysis or facial palsy can be one of the early signs of HIV infection, where the face bends to one side in apparently normal- tensive (with normal BP) individual
3. Growths of the spine and brain tissue
4. Spasm of the blood vessels, constriction of the blood vessel feeding a certain brain area due to hypertension or high blood pressure
5. Clots developing in the heart, in the legs or lungs and going up to block some area of the brain, so called cerebral thrombo –embolism or simply cerebral thrombosis.

Diagnosis-This is where the work of the doctor's hammer is put to proper use, tapping and rubbing! Special brain scan can be very useful, as well as magnetic resonance imaging(MRI), simple blood tests, simple skull x-rays, even registrations of the brain function called Electro Encephalography (EEG)as well as chest x-rays and Electro Cardiograph (ECG) of the heart. Sometimes special Scans are done of blood vessels.

To be honest, the real question always is what can one do with someone who has just had a stroke? Most times since the problem may be deeper in the brain tissue- Nothing, except the usual palliative care. This am afraid has brought many a relative to think their doctors are doing nothing to treat the afflicted. Often strokes are self-limiting, that is if they don't take one's life or sometimes the patient may develop some other complications associated with poor elimination of waste products, eating and mobility. Bed sores for the paralyzed are often frequently met. Strokes may kill as when there is massive bleeding in the brain tissue! If the bleeding is small, the patient especially young ones may completely recover spontaneously.

Something to remember is that the young do much better than the elderly in cases of spontaneous recovery.

47. Malaria

This is one disease that has killed more children than any other in its strides. WHO estimates that more than 500 000 deaths occur annually in Africa related to malaria. Someone once said this is like having a jumbo jet packed full of passengers crashing every hour or less, for a year. The cause of malaria is surprisingly a small bug which resides partly in the mosquito. Someone rightly sad if you doubt that size does not matter, try going to bed with a mosquito! Its buzz is so irritating! Not all mosquitoes can carry malaria. It's carried by the anopheles mosquito common in the tropics.

Types of malaria, according to type of plasmodium. This difference is more theoretical than clinical, in a way. It's quite irrelevant outside the laboratory. Or research facility. As it is, malaria is malaria!

1. Plasmodium Falciparum -the most common in our areas

2.Plasmodium vivax

3.Plasmodium Ovale

4.Plasmodium Malarae. Malaria is a funny disease, it can mimic any condition in the body. Health workers know this very well and those who miss to appreciate this fact lose a lot of patients treating other things when the cause is just malaria.

<u>Symptoms and signs</u>

Common symptoms are fever, headache, body pains, vomiting, diarrhoea, general body pains, loss of appetite, anaemia. Others are fits or convulsions and confusion, jaundice or yellow eyes, kidney failure, low plate counts-when serious.

Diagnosis

Involves a simple blood test in which the parasites malaria plasmodium can easily be seen in the microscope. Sometimes quick tests can be done based on the same principles that HIV test are done-Immunologic tests-testing the presence of anti- bodies in the blood

Complications of malaria are well known. Patients can develop anaemia, jaundice, bleedings, confusion and fits. Death is often a result of such complications, often related to renal or kidney failure and fitting. A person may develop severe anaemia since the parasites destroy the red cells in which they are transported, this can cause thrombocytopenia or low platelets leading to severe bleeding episodes.

Treatment

Anti-malarial drugs are used either orally or in the muscles or veins depending on the severity of the case. We have seen in the recent times malaria has developed resistance to the very common drug, chloroquine that saved us so well over the years. Quinine is still effective for severe or cerebral malaria, albeit with all its antecedent complications of temporary damage to the retina and hearing nerves. Quinine can also on its own cause anaemia or even liver or kidney failure when used in high doses. Patients need to be well hydrated with fluids. Remember, the loss of hearing or sight is a temporary thing that passes away slowly after withdrawing the quinine.

<u>Prevention</u> of malaria is cardinal in its control

-Use of residual spraying of homes and ponds of standing water

-Use of mosquito repellents, fumigating home steads

-Use of mosquito nets. Am told of some fellows who make fishing nets out of donated mosquito nets! A case of choosing to die from malaria on a full stomach of fish!

-Use of preventive drugs as in pregnancy and travellers from malaria devoid areas to malaria infested regions. Travellers needing such prevention should remember to start their drugs at least three weeks before making the trip to a malaria area and continue two to three weeks after leaving the region.

Currently information is reaching us that a vaccine for malaria is undergoing serious tests and has shown promising results

48. Cancer

Since my school days, the definition has not changed. Our professor used to define it as growth minus differentiation. All he was saying is that, this is a condition characterised by uncontrollable aimless growth of tissues involved.

Causes:

1. Largely unknown

2. Viruses as in skin cancer of the Kaposi sarcoma type caused by HPV or a form of human papilloma virus, cervical also caused by another type of HPV.

3. Toxicities like cigarette smoke in lung cancer

4. Damage to bone marrow as in radiation of any nature, as in cases of leukaemia or blood cancers, skin cancers from ultra violet burning

5. Chronic growths transforming into cancer as in fibroids, some times

6. Chronic inflammation of tissue as in stomach cancers. Inflammations can be caused by either viruses, bacteria or toxic substances working in unison or singularly

7. Effects of some "foods" acting on the colon or rectum

The presentations of the complaints will largely depend on the location and extent of damage to concerned organ but can involve pain, tumours or growths, disruption of function, bleeding, blockage of nerves and blood vessels, fits or convulsions, paresis or weakness or even paralyses of a given part or whole limb, failure of several organs

Investigations-Range from simple full blood count, urinalysis, x-rays, scans, CT scans, and microscopic identifications

Treatment can range from drugs (chemo therapy) to irradiation or radio therapy, surgery and palliative measures. It is important therefore to have yearly health examinations of the cervix in child bearing women, breast examinations in all women and prostate cancer tests for men above 40 yrs. of age, chest x rays at regular intervals, though this has its own side effects! Some cancers are easily treatable while others are hardly able to respond to treatment. But don't listen to smooth talkers of miracle reliefs be it from prophets or certain traditional healers. The more time you waste the worse the prognosis or outcome. Spontaneous recovery as in all disease should not be taken as a miracle, in medicine the body is the often the best doctor

49. Epilepsy as a disease

Some Africans believe epilepsy cannot be managed in hospitals. Do not believe them. First things first: Epilepsy is a condition by characterized by repeated fits or seizures or sometimes called convulsions.

Few individuals have never had an episode of fits in their lives. But when such repeats, a diagnosis of epilepsy is established.

There are 3 common types of epilepsy. There is the grand mal epilepsy or the major one, the petit mal epilepsy or the small one and what is generally called absence.

The cause of fits or seizures is all in the biochemical changes or structural changes in the brain. When a large part of the brain is affected, the seizures tend to be major covering the whole body. When it is a small part of the brain affected, it results in fits of the just small areas like a limb or part of the body.

Absence is a kind of epilepsy was the individual involved loses momentarily concentration or consciousness. This is a case like when a child freezes in the middle of taking some notes.

Different factors can lead to seizures, alcohol, haemorrhages or bleeding in the brain, past traumas with scar brain formations, infections like malaria and meningitis. When a defined cause like infection can be identified, this is not called epilepsy. It's more accurate to talk of the reason the person is fitting as diagnosis, than epilepsy.

Diagnosis is a matter of exclusion so to say. Electro encephalography or electrical registration of the brain's activity is often employed in diagnosis to help pick up areas of hyper activity in the brain matter.

An Epileptic fit usually occurs like this; an individual cry out, falls down as in grand mal epilepsy, fitting of the whole or parts of the body, may defecate or pass urine, may bite their tongue. The individual there after enters into a deep sleep, especially if the seizures are major.

Treatment generally is not definite but involves managing the re occurrence of the fits. Sometimes surgery may be helpful but this is often done in very big centres. Anti-convulsant drugs are used to prevent and manage fits. In childhood however, sometimes the condition is self-limiting. The truth is Epilepsy can be managed by health workers.

50. Warts (Condylomata Accuminata) revisited

Warts or some benign growths on the skin or epithelium of a given organ are caused by a virus, human papilloma virus that is the same virus responsible for the development of cervical cancer in women.

Warts easily bleed and rot causing extreme discomfort when too large, they may be secondarily infected.

Warts can be treated by burning or cattery or by use of highly active substances that dissolve the warts such as podophyllin or podotoxin creams. Warts have a propensity to recur even after cautery. There are most aggressive in pregnancy. Remember that Podophyllin/ Podotoxin application in pregnancy is contra indicated and on bare skin can be very corrosive, all the reason why it is usually given under the direction of a health worker.

51. Sickle cell disease

Almost 1 fifth of the population is affected by SCD.

It is a disease characterized by painful joints and fevers brought about by blockages of blood vessels by dying red cells, the Erythrocytes.

It is essentially a heredity disease. It is therefore passed from parent to child. This is a disease where deformed Erythrocytes, take on character of a sickle, hence the name. Normally red cells live for 120 days in the body.

Sickle cells have much shorter lives, their massive break up may clog the vessels and deny them of oxygen. Hence the pains felt in various parts of the body.

Low oxygen or hypoxia leads to pain. SCD is common in areas where there is malaria. It is therefore considered an evolution "mistake" of nature against malaria parasites.

In a crisis of SD blood vessels get occluded, thrombosis or clots are formed. Thus, can lead to chronic ulcers and infections. SCD is a haemolytic disorder, meaning that it is characterized by break up of red cells which carry Haemoglobin that in turn carry oxygen.

It is a disease much more common in Negros, Patients who may suffer from joints, chest pains, and pains. They may develop yellow or jaundiced eyes. Children who are sticklers are often mentally and physically restarted, they may develop deformations in limb as well. They often may not live beyond puberty

Genetic mapping of carriers of sickle cell trait exists but it be common as it is expensive. Unfortunately, children with SCD do not live very long. Few make it to 30 years.

There is no definite treatment except control. Folic acid, vitamin B 12 tablets, are used. Patients are put on anti-malaria prophylaxis. Antibiotic are often used to prevent infections. SCD is indeed a very difficult condition to manage, just like many a hereditary disorder is.

52. Elephantiasis

You have heard about this one. Often there is a lot of misleading information circulating on this disease. Its scientific name is called filiaris. It is caused by a worm, a nematode from a family of filaroid. These worms appear like threads and are particularly prone to attacking the lymphatic system; the lymphatic system is the system that carries lymph, a yellow like substance containing T cells for defence against diseases.

The most common of these worms is Wuchereria Bancroft or Brugia Malayi; the females can grow up to 100 mm while the male can go up to a length of 135 mm. they are transmitted by mosquito bites and once in the body take one year to mature. Elephantiasis got its name from the swollen scrotums and lower limbs that in advanced disease patients present with. Otherwise this disease is a self-limiting one, comes in circles of 5-10 years in a population.

Blood tests taken between 21.00hrs to 2 a.m. is the way to diagnose the disease. Hetrazan or Diethycarbamazine three times daily in tablet form can cure the disease in about a month. Prevention is aimed at mass treatment of population and measures against getting mosquito bites are a must.

53. Nasal Bleeding

"A jug feels drop by drop".

What to do?

1. Pinch the nostrils and hold them tight for 5 minutes. Usually this is enough to stop the bleeding.
2. In a health set up, blow out any blood clots from the nose. Pack the nostrils with gauze dissolved in a mixture of 1ml adrenaline with 10mls of normal saline with a tinge of pain killer drug Novocaine or Lidocaine. Leave the pack in the nostrils for 15 minutes.
3. If the bleeding persists, you may do an anterior pack using Vaseline gauze. Pack the nostrils tightly then check the oval pharynx or upper throat for any posterior nasal bleeding. If there is post nasal bleeding remove the anterior pack, insert a Foley catheter No 16 into the bleeding nose and inflate the bulb with water or saline. Pull the Catheter so that the bulb firmly presses on the inside of the bleeding nose. You may complement this with an anterial (front) pack. Leave packs for 24 hours before removing, provide pain killers and antibiotics. Oxygen and sedation can be given to the patients.

54 Menstrual disorders

Most frequent are increased bleeding and heavy bleeding or memo (metro) rhaggia, painful menses or dysmenorrhea and absence of menses or amenorrhoea. Increased bleeding in a female is often common condition if at persists it's often due to stress or hormonal imbalance.
Growths like fibroids in the womb can also cause women to bleed a lot, as the womb fails to contact adequately to stop the bleeding. The cause of painful periods has not been under stood fully in Gynaecology. What is true is that women with painful periods seem to produce high levels of prostaglandins, a hormone mostly found in smooth muscles.
Treatment of dysmenorrhea is often difficult induce save to say that most episodes resolve spontaneously. An anti-prostaglandin drug like   aspirin taken during menses is usually is beneficial.
As for absence or amenorrhea this usually a condition that comes as a result of aging, a condition called menopause. However, the most frequent cause for absence of menses is of course pregnancy! Stress comes as a second best in as far as amenorrhea is concerned in a woman who suddenly develops missed periods in the absence of pregnancy.
Heavy and prolonged bleeding is often treated with hormones or pills as well as cleaning of the womb with instruments. A test for cancer is always taken to rule it out in child baring women.

---

55. Anaemia

Anaemia or "little blood" can be understood to mean a reduction in red blood cell mass. We all know that the red cells contain a substance called haemoglobin, the substance that helps the cells carry oxygen to different organs in the body.

Red cells are manufactured in the bone marrow and their grave yard is the spleen. A spleen is a pearl shaped organ in the left flank of the abdomen.

Red cells normally live in the body for 120 days, after which new cells new cells are produced from a combination of bile, iron and globin a protein. The whole process being controlled by a chemical from the kidneys called Erythrpoetin. Erythropoetin is a hormone essentially. A hormone is chemicals produced in minute doses in several organs. Examples of hormones we commonly meet in practice are Eostrogen, Progesterone, Thyroxin from the thyroid gland, Adrenaline from the adrenal gland.

So, anaemia then is any reduction due to any reason of the blood cell mass. Common reason for anaemia is bleeding or loss of white blood cells and reduced production of red blood cells. Blood loss can be as a result of heavy menstruation, growth in the womb or fibroids, womb infections, general sickness of a woman whereas increased destruction of red cells can be a result of infection such as malaria, HIV or some virus causing what is called haemolytic (result of break down); this is usually an iron deficiency anaemia. Chemicals or drugs can also lead to reduced destruction of red cells, as well.

Reduced production of red blood cells can be a result of cancer of the bone marrow or blood, lack or reduced red blood vitamins intake (folic acid, B12, Iron etc.) or x ray destruction of the bone marrow.

What is important to remember is that anaemia is never a diagnosis, there is always a cause for it. Anaemia alone does not say much about why the condition is present in the body. So, anaemia is not a disease as such but a sign of a disease   The person with anaemia easily feels tired, appears pale or white, has heart palpitations, develops shortness of breath or experiences fainting episodes as well as headaches. An anaemic person is more prone to develop different infections in the body.

A simple haemoglobin blood estimation is usually carried out to confirm a diagnosis of anaemia, but a lot more complicated investigation is needed to explain the cause for it.

Treatment, therefore, is aimed at the cause. It is therefore, wrong to think that every anaemic patient needs replacement of iron tablets as is often taken for granted by most people. Only the anaemias that are iron deficient types would benefit from a supply of exogenous iron. Some may need other components like folic acid, vitamin B 12 preparations or other drugs. In extreme cases blood is given to correct the problem of anaemia.

56. The Kidney and you

You have one brain, one liver, one stomach.
Why you have two kidneys instead of one is somehow a puzzle, because to tell you the truth you really do not as a human being depend so much on the functions of both kidneys, in the sense that, one can do all right. I know someone will say they are two because of their importance in the body; well than why do you have one brain? And for some people I think two stomachs would be a nice thing, with their affinity to food!

Any way kidneys are a paired organ somewhere in the back, they weigh no more than 150 grams each and are about 10 cm in length. Their main function is to:
-removes toxins from your blood and controls levels of such (urea, creatinine, ammonia, uric acid, etc.)
-control the level of the blood pressure
-participate in making components of blood
-regulate the levels of salts and water in your body.
In short kidneys are but a regulatory -excretory organ of the body.
In short, the kidney is always an organ we aware of only when things are not going on well in the body. Otherwise when our engines are optimally working, few even cares to remember them! This is one organ that does not like messing up with as many a patient will painfully discover when they poison these shy organs. Any toxins after messing up the liver eventually ends up in the kidneys for elimination, and that is when problems may arise! The

kidneys also hate shortage of water or blood; they hate low blood pressure as they can shut off at very short notice without warning!

The diseases you are bound to hear of often are the inflammatory type as in pyelonephritis, glomerulonephritis, or simply nephritis, renal stones, abscesses, cancers and nephritic syndrome characterize by high BP, loss of proteins and swellings. Then the other spectrum you are bound to hear of kidney or renal failures, a condition none of us would like to even test! This is when there is partial or complete shutdown of the function of the kidneys to pump urine. Such patients swell up like footballs, starting with puffy eyes spreading to the whole body! Remember one vital difference with oedema or swelling as a result of the heart which often manifests itself with swollen feet and legs. Oedema or swelling as a result of kidney problems starts from below the eyes! Other than swelling the patient will complain of dull pains in the lumbar parts, passage of scanty urine, bloody urine, urine with pus in it. The thing to remember is never to take any drug you aren't sure of its effect on the kidneys. Kidneys don't like jokes! Kidney diseases can give you headaches, difficulties in breathing, nausea, loss of appetite, dizziness, vomiting, fevers among other complaints.

A simple urine and blood test usually is able to point to problems in the kidneys. But advanced methods range from scans to special x -rays. On average a grown up human takes out about 2 litres of urine daily, which incidentally is the approximate intake of fluids in our bodies daily(with water and food)

Treatment is often aimed at the cause, if it's a drug toxicity mere with draw in time will result in major functional improvement. Other measures are rehydration of the body, control of sugar levels as well as blood pressure. Severe persistent failure may demand direct washing out of blood with a machine called dialysis machine, a very delicate and expensive manoeuvre indeed.

So, look after your kidneys well! Remember that your kidneys are constantly removing toxins in form of urine from your body. It's therefore dis respectful to this humble organ for one to think of detoxifying their bodies by using herbs or tablets! That is a dangerous undertaking which one should avoid!

57. When Pregnancy strays!

Perhaps this condition is only beaten on frequency as a disease for women only by pelvic inflammatory disease (PID). This is a gynaecological condition, called in medical jargon, *'ectopic pregnancy'*, where by a developing foetus grows outside the inside of the womb or uterus. It's often a surgical emergency that requires prompt action in treatment. By type it can be located in either right tube or left. When it sits at the extreme end of the tube is called fimbrial, in the widest area of the tube, it's called ampulla and when it sits in the smallest portion of the tube it's called interstitial. When just by the corners where the tube enters the womb, it's called cornu. Rare locations can be cervical and abdominal or peritoneal.

Though dangerous no woman should die from an ectopic pregnancy once the patient is seen in the health facility. Even when it is missed first time by the attending health worker, it often reveals itself with time. In my thirty years or so of practice in Gynaecology, I Have only seen one death of a woman due to ectopic pregnancy in the hospital! And this case, sorry to say was as a result of extreme callousness on the party of the health workers involved who never reviewed the patient following a missed diagnosis. This patient I recall was left unattended to for several hours during the night. And suffice to say that this case did not happen in our country but in some foreign African country I will not name (lest I open up old wound or wake up a sleeping giant!) Any way the point am trying to make is that this condition though extremely common and dangerous, can easily be managed, the problem may be in recognizing it.

Ectopic pregnancies often occur in women whose tubes have had some form of damage. This damage is often due to untreated STI's or PID, as well as scarring of the tubes by previous surgery on them. Remember that fertilization of the female egg with the male sperm occurs in the tube approximately about the fourteenth day from the first day of the menses; the fertilized product should then ideally be pushed by tubal peristalsis down to the womb for implantation and further growth. Any process which leads to delay of this may lead to the development of an ectopic pregnancy. The tube as you will recall is the size of a ball point inside and can therefore not hold the growing foetus for too long, it then ruptures, leading to severe bleeding and shock of different strengths. We have seen ectopic pregnancies when located in the abdomen growing to near term or even term pregnancies. The developing foetus in this case gets its nourishment from a placenta that forms on the intestines-a very delicate location to handle indeed!

An ectopic pregnancy can when located in the tube be un-ruptured or ruptured, and it is the ruptured ones which present as dire emergencies! The woman can easily pass out from internal bleeding, if left unattended to in just a few hours!

The patient suffering from ectopic pregnancy presents with dull pain in the lower abdominal, if not ruptured and with acute pain, anaemia and extreme tiredness from shock may supervene when it is ruptured-What surgeons call an acute abdomen, closely resembling the pain of a ruptured appendix, only located lower down the abdomen. The pulse will be thready and fast, blood pressure will be low and will keep dropping, all the way to extreme shock state! There will be a period of missed periods but we have seen women who get confused with some bleedings that an ectopic can give when not ruptured which some women may take as a period, there by presenting like no menses were missed. The abdomen is extremely tender to touch and may distend

The diagnosis calls for experience when the ectopic is un-ruptured for it gives very little signs. Whereas when it ruptures, the woman often falls down in extreme pains and is often unable to stand up without help from supporters. An Ultra sound so common ordered by inexperienced staff in ruptured cases is often a worst of valuable time and may be unnecessary, can also be dangerous as it may lead to delays of surgery! When un-ruptured, however it becomes a useful tool in the diagnosis of the problem. An abdominal tap with a needle may reveal non-clotting blood. The cervix of the woman on vaginal examination may give pain when moved from side to side. Bleeding from the woman's private parts may be present but not a must, and when it presents, it's often mild.

A word of caution to health workers here may be in place. Please assume any woman who walks into your consulting room as pregnant till proven otherwise! This way you will avoid the embarrassing misdiagnosis of an ectopic pregnancy that could endanger the health of your patient!

Treatment is easy.it involves cutting out the affected area if in the tube, retying and closing the abdomen after a wash up. This operation in good hands can take just about 15 minutes or less! Suffice to say that its safer done under general anaesthesia as the peritoneum is extremely sensitive to touch when the abdomen is opened. This does not mean life cannot be saved under local anaesthesia if conditions demand it! The treatment of an abdominal pregnancy is beyond the scope of the general public knowledge, so I won't here discuss it.

I can bet my life that once a ruptured tube is tied in an ectopic, the woman rarely requires any transfusion, so common with less experienced health colleagues!

Transfusion of blood has saved lives but it is not without its own dangers especially when carelessly or unnecessarily done. I often told my juniors, "not to transfuse the haemoglobin, but the patient! "Meaning, it's not the levels that matter of the Haemoglobin, but the clinical presentation of the concerned!

Having cautioned about this I truly hope I won't be misunderstood by the Jehovah Witnesses who refuse blood transfusions regardless!

58. You won' t believe it, but it is true!

1. One day I had to do a Caesar while working in Botswana, on a dying mother in the admission ward, in five minutes, with no scrubbing up, with instruments taken from theatre, with no anaesthesia on the patient, we saved the life of the baby but as we had expected the mother was half dead, and she died within seconds of arrival in the maternity ward. She had had cerebral malaria which was badly treated at her home by healers! I think no reported surgery to save a child has ever been done in the admission ward anywhere in the world. This was a first!
We had to do the unconventional so as to save at least the baby. We later looked after the baby in the ward till it was four yrs. old, with my team of nurses that included three Zambian nurses, and then handed over the child to some old relatives!

2. Our head of medicine, Specialist Physician, a white man in one of the hospitals in Botswana was once attacked by the town's people alleging that lumber puncture had been killing patients at the hospital. Little did they know that the cause of deaths had been late admissions to hospital after trying several traditional healings at their homes! The Ministry Of Health had to come very hard in defence of the doctor but he was almost killed!

3. In one small district hospital I worked, my colleague a Kenyan doctor admitted one villager with swollen tummy, An x-ray revealed he has had a bicycle pump inserted thru his anus up to the intestines in order to so called cleanse his colons! The traditional healer then failed to retrieve it, we had to take him to theatre and went in after anaesthetising him and pulled it out with our hands thru the very anus!
Again we checked the medical history on the net, this was a first-insertion of a bicycle pump into someone in order to treat them! Fortunately for the patient he had no damage to the colons!!
Many such bizarre real medical stories you can read in my book available on amazon.com, Confessions of a doctor". Also available by ordering from self. This world can amaze you!

59. Homosexuality-to allow or not to allow, that's the question...

Now before we confuse each other, answer the following questions as honestly as you can...

1.Would you allow your child or brother, sister to be gay or lesbian?

2. Would you allow yourself to be gay or lesbian?

3. If your grandparents were gay or lesbian, would you be reading this?

4. If you grew up in the village, did you hear (or suspect) any of the villagers being gay or lesbian?

5. When did you first become aware of gay /lesbian issues? And from whom?

6. Why do you think almost all whites, including Christians think gays and lesbians should be allowed to marry?

7. Why do you think the African society has not by and large accepted same sex marriages?

8. Do you think a Christian can allow same sex marriages?

9. If you are a believer do you think God allows same sex marriages?

10. Are you gay or lesbian yourself? If so why, if not why?

11. Does biology play dice?

12. Would you allow incest, bestiality or that men marry animals, if yes; why, if not; why?

13. Would you allow women to marry animals? Why and why not?

14. Would you allow your cow or dog to mount its type?

Now the facts
-The first country to allow same sex marriages was Netherlands, followed by Belgium, then Spain, and Canada
-RSA was the first country in Africa and only one to date that allows same sex marriages
-RSA became the number five in the world(1996) to allow same sex marriages
-Donald Trump is against same sex marriages, Obama allowed it
-Not all states in America allow same sex marriages
-Uganda and some Muslim countries have the stringiest laws against same sex relationships in the world
-More educated people are likely to allow same sex marriages as compared to uneducated ones
-Those in towns are more likely to tolerate gay and lesbians and are more likely to be so, as compared to villagers
-The more exposed a society is to western culture, the more likely it is to tolerate gays and lesbians

The Argument from Nature-Some scientists think that gays and lesbians are born that way. That they cannot help their situations. Some think that there is a gene responsible for "gays "and lesbianism, while others think that the brains of gays, the brain centre for sex, is bigger in gays and lesbians. One such scientist postulating the role of nature in this is Dean Hamer-he believes it's genetic! The opponents to gene theory point out that since gays and lesbians do not produce, there was no way they could pass on their genes to their off springs!

The Argument from human rights-Some feel that as long as gays and lesbians do their thing in the confines of their homes, they should not be discriminated against. They argue that gays and lesbians do not harm anybody!
The Argument from nurture-Another group of scientists feel that homosexuality is a learned behaviour. They believe like Emmanuel Kant, a German philosopher of the last century, that man ought to behave in a way that his behaviour may become a universal law. They argue that homosexuality is caused by broken relations in early childhood, that these are often individuals with a dominant single parent, say a mother with an absent or inattentive father...They argue that as a child is growing there is disturbed adaptation to the opposite sex.

60. Cervical Cancer Is Not About Women!

Many men do not want to hear about cancer of the cervix. They feel that it's a disease of women! But read on and see why we all should be interested in preventing this type of cancer.
1. Understanding-Let us start with defining (if we can) the word "cancer". Cancer refers to any uncontrolled growth of any tissue or organ of the body. One of my professors used to call it growth without differentiation or simply put Cancer=Growth-differentiation. In this case we can understand differentiation as a specific target and aim, limited in time and space. Therefore, cells that continue

to multiply beyond limit, chaotically, with no particular aim in sight can be said to be cancerous.

Cervical cancer attacks the neck of the uterus or neck of the womb.

2. In Zambia today cancer of the cervix happens to be the leading cause of deaths among all the cancers such us uterine, prostate, penile, throat, lung, liver, lung, kidney, colon, skin, blood cancers. And the reason is simple, its slow growth in a place hidden from site, in a place that many regard as private, could be the reason why it is often noticed early enough. Am reminded of a case that shocked many some time ago when my colleague, a Gynaecologist, a very prominent women surgeon indeed, a man who saved many women with cancer ended up losing his own wife to the disease without him even being suspicious that the cervical cancer was slowly" eating away" his own wife! By the time he realized the process had become advanced and no one could save her! So now you can understand how secretive this cancer can be!

3. Cause-This is one cancer that has undergone tremendous changes in our understanding of the cause. Whereas 15 yrs. ago or slightly more years ago, we all thought that this cancer attacked those women who had numerous deliveries, who had traumatic changes on the cervix as in repeated abortions and cleaning of the womb, to above 45 yr. olds, we have now revised our understanding that this cancer is an STI/STD. Cancer of the cervix is a sexually transmitted infection! This I should admit I didn't know when I first started treating women in the late 80' s and am not afraid to say so because we simply did not have the information we do today! Who

would have known that the source of the cancer is actually men! And in fact, even the age group at risk has been revised to include all sexually active woman of any age! Cancer of the cervix, as one of my friends like to put it, has grown younger! For me I once attended to and lost a 26-yr. old young woman to cancer of the cervix and am sure my colleagues can vouch that indeed we are increasingly seeing young women afflicted with this disease.

Men have everything to do with cancer. Men harbour the Human Papilloma virus on their sexual organs, more especially the skin that surround the penile head, the prepuce. For this reason, removal of the prepuce in man, respectively called circumcision, may actually reduce the spread of the cancer in women. Not that a circumcised man cannot harbour the Papilloma virus in his penile sweat glands, he can, but the chances are drastically reduced. Same goes with HIV infection whose transmission can be reduced by as much as 40% in circumcised men. Therefore, some face book specialists, who I have read, sometimes pouring scorn on the rationale of circumcision in men in reducing HIV and cancer, often are missing the real issues in transmission of these conditions. This is not to say that you won't find doctors in this world who still can argue and still do argue against the need for male circumcision. That is the beauty of science, consensus on any topic often takes time! Women at risk therefore are those with multiple sexual partners and those women who start too early involving themselves in sexual acts (when the cervix and vagina are rather very easily bruised!) Women with low immunity for one reason or the other are also at a greater risk of developing cancer of the cervix The HPV itself can sit harmlessly in man for years without causing any symptoms. Sometimes though some men may develop warty growths.

4. Early signs —Cancer of the cervix remains unnoticed for many yrs... Its first presentation is often what we call spotting during sexual act or bathing from the woman involved. This is what is called as contact bleeding. This sometimes is wrongly interpreted by the sufferer or some inexperienced health worker as hormonal disturbance related. There is no pain in the abdomen in this early stage!

4. Late complaints-More bleeding episodes , anaemia, smelly discharge and pain as the process spreads further around the abdomen and surrounding organs, producing pressure symptoms(constipation, disturbed urine out flow)as it presses on neighbouring organs including nearby nerve centres, especially the so called nervous plexus, a conglomeration of nerves deep in the abdominal cavity(the cervix itself has no pain receptors, it only responds to pressure).The cancer can spread up wards and down wards to the vagina, it often affects the liver, lungs and the brain, the so called fourth stage of the disease

   Diagnosis-A pap smear or cervical smear is the most important in identifying the deranged cells in the cervix early. This can be done under clinical set ups in a matter of few minutes. Further confirmation can be done by cutting away a small tissue of the cervix for laboratory investigations. This we call in medical parlance, a biopsy.

In developed countries all sexually active women are made to under routine pap smears every year or two. Something we should be thinking about in our developing countries. Vaccinations against the HPV are available nowadays, though a bit on the expensive side!

6. Treatment is simple when caught early. It may involve rubbing the cervix with very active substances, cautery or burning off small areas involved, cutting out portions of the cervix, whole cervix and sometimes whole cervix and uterus, and close by lymph nodes, as well as ovaries. Radio therapy is often resorted to as an adjunct to treatment or as the only means of prolonging some woman's life in late cases.

Please remember to encourage your men and boys to get circumcised and for all sexually active women to undergo Papanicolaou (cervical smears) smears at least once in two years. if not a year

61. Panic Attacks

Who has never suffered from one of these attacks? It is estimated that almost 1/3 of all humanity suffers from this disorder from time to time. This is often a condition that affects young women and can carry within families. We can define it as an exaggeration from response of the body our histories anxiety reaction to the surrounding or events.

The person suffering panic attack out of the blues feels terrible, shaky, hot, develops heart plantation's, feels suffocated and may actually feel sick without often a physical basis, In panic attacks, the hormone adrenaline, the fright hormone so to say is produced in high quantities. Adrenaline as we all know can cause heart partitions and feeling of frights or anxiety. Families with histories of depressive illness or anxieties in their parents are at a great risk of developing panic disorders.

Factors that have a profound effect on panic attacks are the increased intake of caffeine and a strong family history of depressive disorders. Chronically it manifests itself as phobias or fears of heights, animal phobia or fears of animals, phobias of heights etc. what is more surprising is that these reactions do not have an obvious physical cause. They happen out of the blue!

 Approach...Patients are forced to learn to relax, to breath slowly when faced with certain phobia circumstances, they are told to avoid caffeine, avoid solitude. At times hypnotherapy may
Panic attacks

Terms
1. Phobias- Fear and cause
2. Stress- syndrome characterized by chronic miss-adoption
3. Panic attack- exaggerated reaction to the surrounding
-occurs out of the blue
-no cause can be physically determined
Statistics:
1.   Affects 1/3 of humanity
2.   Mostly Women
3.   Affects mostly young people
The reaction of the body in panic attack:

1. Red alert- like a warning takes place of danger in the environment
2. Production of high levels of the fright hormone adrenalin
3. Get away-the body prepares to rum way, so to say
Clinically:

1. BP increases-heart plantations/sick hot flushes/shaking of the concerned individual
2. Pulse increases
3. Sweating, feeling of collapse may have fits, fell like suffocating.
1. Cognitive therapy
2. De-catastrophizing
3. Breathing exercise
4. Aromatic therapy (with rosemary oils)

Self help

1. Relax
2. Breath slowly
3. Auto suggestions/hypnosis

All these may be helpful severally or individually

62. Zika Virus

- Female mosquito transmitted, the Argyti mosquito
- Stays 14 days in mosquito bodies
- 1st isolated in Uganda
- Was also seen in Senegal and Latin America
- No vaccine yet developed

Prevention

- 2-7 days after   the bite-symptoms one in four people to develop symptoms, such as fever symptoms, rash, joint pains, red eyes,
- Mosquitoes lay their Larva-on water
- Off springs with Micro-encelophaly or small heads are often a manifestation of the disease
- Condoms can prevent Zika virus if used correctly, as it is asexually transmitted infection.

28 countries so far affected, including Spain with a patient who first travelled to Colombia.

Zika virus was discovered in the Zika forest- Uganda.

Related: dengue, yellow fever, west Nile viral disease

63. The truth about vitamins

You have probably swallowed multi vitamins before with a view to improve your appetite but truth is such action is often a placebo effect than physically scientific! Your appetite may improve not because of your packet of vitamins but because your mind was meant to believe so! That's what we call placebo effect. This is the same method some prophets use unknowingly or knowingly to make those limping to walk straight! The thing is, when the mind is up to it, even water can treat you!

We call reduced condition of vitamins in your body hypo or simply when they are "lacking " -avitaminosis. Vitamins are minute substances in your body which regulate and act on your metabolism, they help in the growth of cells, and they help in making your body stand up to infections. They do this thru equally smaller substances we shall call enzymes (which themselves are essentially vitamins!)

Where do you get vitamins from?

1. From outside the body or exogenous

2. From inside the body-Endogenic as we call it, mostly from absorptions from the stomach and intestines or from the work of intestinal bugs or microbes. This is, however often not enough is, the body needs to get extra vitamins from outside with the food.

Your body uses more vitamins during infections, during pregnancy (you recall, we always give folic acid), during breast feeding and during heavy or delicate mental work.

These vitamins may be damaged by over cooking of food, in instances of liver disease, or in cases of use of cortico-steroids like hydrocortisone, and may go down when antibiotic drugs are used for longer periods. In rare circumstances, you may have a condition of heightened quantities, or hyper vitaminosis, with especially vitamins like D, and A, the so-called fat-soluble vitamins along with vitamin E, and K. The other vitamins dissolve easily in water such as vitamin C, B, and P (So called water soluble vitamins)

1. Vitamin A deficiency-May lead to poor vision during night time, greying and dropping of hair, anaemia and a whole lot of upper respiratory inflammatory diseases.
You get vitamin A from liver, egg yolk, butter, carrots, tomatoes, apricots, lettuce and spinach
for this reason you now are hearing of vitamin A fortified mealie meal and other foods. But am also aware that we have started giving children, all children some vitamin A preventative drops at birth. Just shows how important this vitamin is to the body.
2. Vitamins group B's-Quite numerous types. Deficiency may lead to problems in the central nervous system and heart and various mouth problems like stomatitis or inflammations...B1 deficiency is causes a condition we call Beri Beri, which presents with swellings of limbs, constipation, passing of wind, pain in limbs etc.
Foods- giving vitamin B groups are wheat products, pork, potatoes, and peas, liver

3. Vitamin PP or Nicotinic acid. Deficiency causes a condition we call pellagra characterized by the three D-

Dementia, Diarrhoea and Dermatitis. Sources are proteins.

For some reason the name Vitamin PP is rather very uncommon among our students in Zambia, most use the term Nicotinic acid, but it is one and the same thing!

4. Vitamin K-Very useful in controlling bleeding. This one is given at birth as injection to all the babies.

5 Vitamin C or Ascorbic acid- Always a vital vitamin found in fruits and veggies, very essential in the absorption of iron in the stomach, very helpful in improving wound healing and development of resistance to infections. Deficiency is called Scurvy characterized by haemorrhages and loose teeth, bleeding gums, rapid fatigue and general weakness

Well these are some of the more important vitamins. We can't discuss all in this page, suffice to say that the best source of vitamins is always food, not tablets!

64. Insomnia

Otherwise called lack of adequate sleep or simply lack of sleep.

No one can claim that they have never tossed and turned in bed with wide open eyes, never falling asleep but when this becomes repeated over a period of time, it then becomes insomnia! How do you resolve lack of sleep?

1. Take meals at late hours that are easy to absorb

2. Avoid taking such drinks as dragons, red bull, or other high containing caffeine beverages at least not less than 4 hours before you sleep! These are usually used by people wanting to stay awake and alert, longer, like long distance drivers or students. Over time, your body will demand higher and higher doses, more frequent doses, or you just get addicted!

3 When you are tired take a nap, don't push your body to extremes or take a break, go for some fresh air, take a walk, listen to some classic music.

4. Avoid watching horror movies just before you sleep, they may turn up in your dreams!

5. Avoid quarrels with your spouse before bed time, or with yourself! Learn to accept situations you can't change and change those you can!

6 If in pain take pain killers, but they have to be safe. Avoid aspirin if you have ulcers or gastritis

7.Avoid sleeping remedies like Valium, they eventually turn you into a slave who won't sleep without them, they may have adverse health effects if taken over long periods, or in high doses! Or even harm your liver!

8. If you are stressed ask for counselling, if you can't

resolve the issues yourself. If you are afraid of chronic diseases, ask for counselling.

9. Sleep in a mosquito net or use insect repellents, or simply "doom "up your room well before bed time

10. Avoid sleeping with braziers on (*mbabula*), they are a source of carbon monoxide, which has no smell but can make your night the last! Here, it's more than insomnia!

11 Avoid wrecking your traditional sleeping hours because of late studies! Schedule your work long before midnight!

12 Avoid thinking of "lost" lovers, relatives, husbands, wives, children, colleagues, before you go to sleep...they are gone, you won't change a thing!

This list is not conclusive!

65. Male Circumcision-Get the facts!

1. Involves cutting away the prepuce of the male organ

2. If your work involves long periods of lack of water to bathe, it does promote hygiene-like soldiers on ops. Duties in the bushes, long distance drivers etc.

3. Reduces possibility of transmission of HIV to your partner, reduces the chances of getting infected by the same as the most pliable piece of your male organ is no longer there. The possibility of getting micro cuts during sexual act, is reduced by far

4. Can be done in very small children without any prolonged discomfort

5. In Adults can be done under local anaesthesia in less than 10 minutes

6 Sensations are reduced but only minimally so, often it's more psychological than physical!

7. Sometimes when done by inexperienced hands can lead to bleeding and infection. But heals within seven-10 days under normal circumstances.

8. Reduces chances of transmission of human Papilloma virus or HPV by 30-40% to your female partner. Note cervical cancer in the female is caused by HPV, reduces chances of getting infected and passing on the infection of STI's

Male circumcision is not organ mutilation, as no permanent damage with terrible repercussions is done to the male organ. However, it's not a 100 % method to prevent disease and should therefore be done or not done with full knowledge of the pros and cons!

66. Basic understanding of fractures

Loosely can be understood as a break in the continuation of the bone architecture or structure.
Am aware that this problem is often misunderstood and sometimes badly treated. The facts are thus:
Causes of fractures;
1. Accidents of different types, falling or being hit by a vehicle, or thru sports activities.
2. Pathological fractures-often this happens in older people without any undue stress as the bones in such people do tend to lose their strength (de -mineralization). In kids up to Primary school going age the site is often the wrist and above the elbow (supracondylar fractures).
Blood vessels are elastic and often escape damage, nerve branches are often small and regrow slowly if given time.
What to expect:
Any fracture if left alone can actually heal, and does heal! The only problem is it may take much longer time and perhaps leave a deformation as the fragments are not well aligned. We have seen this in animals which accidentally break their bones-the fracture do heal.

The other thing is, all bones have blood supply, so there could be bleeding. We know, for example, that pelvic fractures can bleed up to 2 litres of blood which may be not manifest to the outside if the skin is intact over the bones. This can cause extreme shock and sometimes if not corrected in time can lead to death.
Spinal fractures are particularly dangerous with disruption

of function and sensation of the organs lower down the fracture site. For this reason, when you find someone in an accident, the best you can do is to avoid moving them about without medical assistance! This I have seen has led to many complications in accident victims in our country! The blood pressure by some reflex mechanism is always dropping in spinal fractures!

Simple fractures- treatment;

-arm sling on the arm to prevent pain by movement

-pain killers are given

-bleeding is stopped by pressure or temporary tying (not more than 2 hrs.!) on the limbs

-Then you can have a plaster of Paris fitted or an operation with "nails" to fix the bones is done in a health facility. This is rarely necessary in kids!

-The arm sling or POP (Plaster of Paris) is kept for three to six weeks in kids, and a bit longer in adults. Nails inserted in adults can be later be removed after healing or left in the bone.

Remember bones heal on their own, so long the fragments are not too far off, and so there is nothing to panic about!

Rib fractures do not need any particular treatment, other than controlling pain! Whereas fractures of the skull bones and face may also be left untouched if they do not lead to too much bleeding into the head, or are not protruding too much down wards to the brain tissue. Fractures in the leg can be treated for as long as six months or more, but such people often start to move as soon as pain is controlled. Therefore, be wary of prophets who claim all sorts of things vis a vis treating of fractures.

These people often operate on your ignorance that fractures do heal, if left alone with time!
Fractures in the feet, toes and hands often don't need any particular manipulation, other than controlling pain.
Finger fractures may be treated with only bandages or some simple splinting.

67. Talent is not inherited!

Sounds pretty crude statement to make, but it may just be true!
Check this-why are there more discoveries and inventions in Europe, China and Russia and less so in Southern America, Africa and the greater Asia?
-Why Hillcrest and DK Secondary schools been so dominant with getting first class results in Zambia? Is it the material they get raw, or it's the culture present at these schools that continues to churn out geniuses! Is it that these schools have better facilities inherited from the colonialists or the kids are just smart? Or do they get different better teachers?
-Why are generations of Brazilians from the times of Pele to Neymar so dominant in football (Brazil has won the world cup 5 times)?
-Why are African Americans so good at boxing, basketball and volleyball, sprinting?
-Why are Russians so dominant in chess? Indians in cricket? Kiwis in rugby? Are they special people?

-why this and not that? Why?

Why are African ladies so poor at maths and don't like engineering studies?

Can we call a girl doing, badly at Arithmetic dull naturally when the same girl can speak Japanese, Chinese or Vietnamese, Bemba. Lozi, Tonga?

Unless we can recognize that we are all born geniuses (well with a few real idiots!) we shall pretty well continue to wallow in poor results and underdevelopment.

Give me any child at three yrs. old and I can make it into a Grand master at chess! Give me a child at 3 yrs. old, and I can create a music genius! A Bob Marley! Give me a child at three yrs. I can make it play football like Messi or Maradona, I can make it into a nuclear scientist like Albert Einstein! I can make a Stephen Hawking from any child!

Why are the Ayew Brothers football greats in Ghana following their Dad's (Abedi Pele) footsteps? Why are the Musonda boys doing so well in Holland football? Why not the Kalusha ones? Why are the Williams' sisters so good in tennis, were they born like that? Ask Mr. Williams, he created their talent by simply teaching and guiding them at an early age!

It's all in training and not in born traits!!I put it to you, that nature pretty gives all of us almost the same limitless capacity of brain, some just don't have the chance to develop it, grow it, use and improve on it! Any talent can be trained thru proper education and guidance! That nature lazy *bums* blame for their situation can be nurtured! Nature needs to be nurtured!

Maybe we should tailor our education to what we really

want to have in Society?
No, talent I say it again is not inherited! Do you agree?

68. Why HIV isn't a biological weapon!

1. It cuts across all nations, poor, and rich, some less affected than others but affected all the same.
2. A biological weapon would need to have some form of storage, such storage should not change the virility or strength of the weapon
3. Such a weapon has to have mass destructive tendencies in a short period of time to make any impact, not yrs.! HIV takes yrs. to develop into Aids, sometimes not even always!

4. The delivery weapon would not be thru sex mainly as the front line of fighting soldiers rarely engage in mass sexual acts! Neither can HIV be delivered thru a bomb!

5 A biological weapon to be effective must spread very fast and be difficult to stop or control. HIV is easily stopped by abstinence and use of condoms!

6. A weapon like that must be very difficult to trace. HIV is simple to diagnose!

7. A biological weapon such as anthrax germs and some nerve agents are known to stay long outside the body of a human or can easily spread thru the atmosphere. HIV when exposed outside the human blood (cell) does not survive more than 10 minutes at the most!
Please stop the conspiracy theories circulating that HIV is a weapon aimed at blacks! Hope you have listened!

69. Blood groups and Parentage

Have you wondered if that child is yours?
The surest way, the most expensive is a DNA test, it is never wrong nor doubtful. Many do not have the benefit of doing a DNA test. The simplest, which at least can give you the possibilities is by doing blood groups of yourself, the child and your partner. Note this is not conclusive but can at least give you what is not possible.
There four blood groups, followed by a specific factor called Rhesus factor. Rh or Rhesus factor is an anti-gene on the red cells, this what gives you the negative or positive end of your blood group. You have, A Positive and A negative positive and B negative, AB positive and AB negative. Negative blood groups are rare, about 15 % of people, the rest are all positive. Negative groups to avoid genetic disease have to marry only negative groups! If this type of person marries a positive partner, they run the risk of the baby dying in the womb or being born sick!
So any way if you are A and your partner is B, and vice versa, the child can only be, if it's yours either A, B, or AB,

never group 0, unless such group O is out of a double recessive gene 0.If on the other hand you the "parents" are both Group 0, you can't have a child with Group A, B, or AB !if on the other hand you are both AB, you can have a child with A, B, or AB, never Group 0!This here is a simple self-screening you can do , to check out the possibilities!

70. Coma

All health workers know the creepy feeling when they are called or receive a patient in coma, especially if this patient be a child, with no relatives or parents to give what happened immediately before the child became comatose. This is hell on earth, trying to unravel this one! Student doctors or interns "hate" comatose patients so do nurses nursing such, precisely because all the book knowledge seems to jump out of the window on this one! Older doctors " hate" comatose patients for then the poor fellows are called to assess such cases at very odd hrs. Post-midnight especially. It can take hrs. And by the time one goes back to sleep, one is supposed to be reporting back to work!

However the good doctors know one thing for sure that the problem is located in the brain. It's always the brain, what else? One then has to start thinking fast of what can lead to this unresponsiveness (coma) in a patient.

For the common man out there, keep well away trying to

unravel and over do things, trying to help this patient. We would appreciate, if all you did is keep them from danger, you don't put anything in the mouth forcefully and you turn them to the side-We shall surely thank you for this! Then the other harder part starts we look at the possibility of trauma to the head by falling or motor car accident. We look for external signs on the head, any marks or swelling? Or could it be that the person is simply had too much to drink? Or are they epileptic or diabetic, mad?

Or perhaps it is severe malaria, meningitis, brain abscess, typhoid fever, cancer in the head, stroke following high BP? Dehydration leading to severe loss of fluids? Or that the person has taken dangerous medications, overdose? Or maybe it's a complicated pneumonia, TB, Liver disease or renal failure or is it septicaemia (generalized infection of the body from a different source within the body)? Or maybe someone has had sudden bleeding from a burst vessel in the head, an aneurysm? Or, or, your brain get jammed!

Could the patient be pregnant and had fitted (you become a *Gyno* or maternity doctor by implication!)

Coma can be so confusing that the inexperienced panicky dr. even gets more confused in the process! No one wants a patient to die during their call or in their hands-you get the sense?

So a quick smell of the nose is done-alcohol? A quick sugar is done, a full blood count, an x-ray here and there, or perhaps you going to need to do a quick lumber puncture (the relatives say no? Now you get really mad...and

sometimes you draw a blank Cheque! What are you going to tell the relatives, your senior, busy snoring at home? Please feel for the poor doctor when faced with a comatose patient, feel for the nurse who has to turn your patient every two hrs., feed them thru the tubes or monitor the drips throughout the night, while having the conscious ones permanently calling' 'nurse! Nurse!"
It's a crazy world this medicine! And for the doctors to be confronted by their waste nightmare, the high-ranking politician breathing on their necks', doctor what's is wrong with my niece? Can we, help, perhaps phone the President?" Jesus, you just get even madder, what the hell is the President going to do with a comatose patient!

71. Masturbation-The Truth

First the basics of sexuality in man and woman...
Sex is a product of a fertile mind, it happens in the mind. Boys or men do have wet dreams in which they become erotically aroused in a dream and actually come off! This normally happens when a boy or man, who is sexually active, has had a big break before engaging in sex. The body is clever, it has a way of self-cleansing using the subconscious mind. When a boy, girl, woman or man consciously brings oneself to orgasm thru different means, this is what is called masturbation (self-stimulation to orgasm). The satisfaction according to the body, the brain, is the same as the actual sexual act.

So then how does a normal sexual response become unhealthy? Unless of course in rare circumstances, the man or woman takes conscious steps to replace for good the mode of sexual gratification, and then want to change to the real act after a long time. Perhaps one could then talk of minor psychological difficulties, but such cases are as rare as snow in summer!
In few words masturbation has no dangers to health!

72. Contraceptives

Here is a rough guide to failure rates of different contraceptives...
So long from the outset, you do understand that the final decision which method would be best is always an individual decision, after discussing the pros and cons with your health worker. No method is/ has a100% success rate, other than, of course, abstinence!
I will rate the methods in a descending manner from the poorest to the strongest.
Now, this number is from a one yr. of use and relates to the number of those from a 100 women using the method that would get pregnant.
1.No method-70
2.Douching, rhythm method or what you call "danger days '' method-30
3.Coitus interrupts(when the male with draws as he is about to ejaculate-25
4.Foams, creams, jellies, vaginal suppositories-15
5.cervical cap-13

6. diaphragm with spermacide-13

7, The "famous" condom-10

8.intra uterine devices(loops)-4

9 mini pill (this contains Progestorone only)-3

10. combined pill (Microgynon, Eugynon, Ovrall, Overette etc)- 2

11.injectables(like Depo Provera)- 0.25

12.Vasectomy(male tying)- 0.15

13, Tubal ligation (female tying of tubes)-0.04.

From the above, it follows that tying tubes of women is the most successful method, after abstinence! I hope this clarifies the so many questions we got on contraceptives!

73. Pregnancy tips

1. Always register for Ante natal clinic (ANC)

2. Every pregnancy has its own tale, do not think you should have had the problem before, when it occurs in your present one

3. Swelling of feet (oedema) is not an ominous sign if not accompanied by changes in BP and proteins in urine.it does not need any treatment but just assurance. Never use drugs that push out water (diuretics) in treating simple oedema!

4. Hypertension in pregnancy must be aggressively addressed, especially if there are proteins in urine (kidney involvement). Progressive rises in BP and proteins in urine

in spite of treatment may call for termination or delivery of the pregnancy, regardless of gestation period!

5, Pregnancy may change your food preferences, but eating soil should be discouraged! Soil may contain eggs for worms and may contain very dangerous germs, sometimes.

6 The dictum "once a Caesar, always a Caesar", is an old women's tale, it's not true!

7. No drug is completely safe in pregnancy, except water! It's a matter of weighing the risk Vis a Vis the benefit

8. Other than iron, folic acid, no supplements are necessary in pregnancy

9. There is always a drop in the haemoglobin levels in any pregnancy, but it should not be too high. The reason is that there is haemo- dilution (blood dilution) with increased fluid in any pregnancy

10. Diabetes in pregnancy, pregnancy induced hypertension and Iso-immunisation (ABO, blood group incompatibility) should never ever be taken up to term for delivery. Delivery must be effected by 37 weeks gestation by the most appropriate means.

74. Ultra -Sound or Scanning in pregnancy

Have you ever wondered why some times your request to have a scan in pregnancy at your own time may not be entertained by midwives and doctors? Any investigation is as good as the information it can provide.
A woman would normally have three scans in the nine months barring any problems.
1. Before 12 weeks or three months, a scan is indicated for localization of the pregnancy and determining gestation period or expected date of delivery. Sometimes used to see if the gestation sac is intact, the number of sacs may be well defined (twins or not)

2. 20 weeks-24 weeks (the period when late abortions can be entertained. Here the organs of the baby are well defined-the spine, the kidneys, the heart. Neuro abnormalities or any other abnormalities can easily be seen. The position of the foetus is immaterial, as it swims in a pool of liquor (water, not alcohol!) and may change position as often as it wants. Expected date of delivery is well defined by the scan. Investigations like amniocentesis, the study of the state of liquor and indirectly foetus are often may be done. Placental location is often irrelevant to continued care, as there is no labour!
Sex determination of the baby is possible but often not an indication to demand a scan (unless of course you are Indian, who culturally we are told may loathe female foetuses). In Zambia, one would think it's an irrelevant

issue, as you can do very little about it, am told you have unisex clothes early in life!

3 After 37-38 weeks to plan mode of delivery as placental position won't change, the size of baby changes little, the position in the womb is fixed. The amount of liquor and condition or activity of the foetus is documented. Size of baby is automatically measured. One thing though size should be relative to maternal pelvis!

75. Penicillin revolutionised medicine!

When George Bush went after Saddam Hussein in Iraq many people got injured in battle. Without the use of penicillin during surgeries like amputations and abdominal injuries many could have kicked the bucket!
Penicillin happens to be the first naturally occurring agent that turned the world of infections upside down. Accidentally discovered by a Lab Technician working on the flu virus, Sir Alexander Fleming. This drug has made us treat Gonorrhoea, syphilis, endocarditis (inflammation of the "inside" of the heart), meningitis, pneumonia which previously would kill people in -mass. Fleming discovered this drug from a mould that grew accidentally on a growth of bacteria in his lab in London.
Now for those getting all excited about how plants can give you medicines, read this...
1. He was a lab technician, not a lawyer, already studying diseases!
2. He was working in a well-equipped lab in London
3. His medicine only knew wide spread use after 1942! He

discovered it in 1928!
4. Laboratories had to come in with scientists to work out extraction of the active ingredient, the doses and the like
5. Fleming did not use anecdotes of successes to convince the world!

76. The Tongue as a window!

I recall one of my professors saying that he could tell you about your health by looking at your tongue. I thought he was a big joke, but having practiced close to three decades, the old fellow was right! I believe what his old brain was hinting as i joined him with white hair!
1. White tongue or pale one-shows you have anaemia or little blood
2. A red tongue may show you have too much blood or red blood cells
3 A yellow coat -would show liver derangement or infection like malaria or inflammation of the liver-hepatitis or even a liver cancer-Hepatoma or your gall bladder output may be blocked by a stone or growth in its ducts.
4. A white coat- May suggest a digestive problem
5.A dry tongue may suggest dehydration
6. A geographic tongue, with lines like a map, though people might think is a problem actually does not mean a thing!

77. Iatrogenic illnesses

I know experience is the best teacher! Nothing beats experience!

Most people know, except perhaps prophets, it's a sobering thought that most sick people in fact do recover without any treatment at all. Health workers know this very well, that's why sometimes they give you worthless medications (but harmless ones) knowing very well you will recover. Some people may think and attribute this to miracles but the truth is, the body is always the best doctorr!

Sometimes some people think injections heal better than tablets, also not exactly true. Just like the feeling that the bitter the medications, the better it is! This is often used by traditional healers to their advantage!

So Iatrogenic illnesses are the ones healers bring about to you in their search for "better treatments" that may not have a medical basis, or sometimes side effects of doing too much of anything as relates to investigations and treatment strategies that may be undertaken by a health worker. Which cases come to mind?

1. Tonsillectomy (removal of tonsils)-I will surprise you, this operation is often unnecessary. Apart from the tragedy of those who actually die from the operation, there is no evidence, am afraid, to show that the survivors derive any benefit that might compensate the bereaved!

2. Intravenous fluids or what in Zambia, we call "drips". Drips, you might want to know carry risks. Of course, the benefits of drips far outweigh the dangers but a wrong electrolyte not indicated can cause a lot of damage, all the

way to over loading the heart and lungs! Or an infection can be introduced thru the skin to the body!

3 X /ray-Please don't force your way to getting unnecessary x rays, it could be the difference for a future cancerous growth in years to come. Or it could affect your fertility! Let me add that to do an x ray when not indicated is negligent, but also not to do an x/ray when it is indicated is also negligent!

4 Tongue tie- The cutting of the supposed tongue tie in a talking child is a misnomer of treatment, Tongue ties do not really exist, except for the grandmothers!
Let me close by saying that health workers have always to ask themselves whether the treatment or investigations they order on a patient are really necessary or they aren't. This is the only way to avoid iatrogenic illnesses.

78. Multi-Drug Resistant TB (MDR-TB)

What is it?
Normally all TB is treatable, but when it is resistant to the two common drugs normally used to treat it-Isoniazid and Rifampicin. TB germs become resistant when they cannot be eradicated effectively in spite of treatment. The symptoms for this type of TB is however the same as the normal TB and can only be confirmed by lab tests.

How does one get it?
1. Stopping treatment before being told to do so-most

people with TB feel better two weeks after starting treatment for TB and therefore may feel like stopping the drugs on their own, before in reality all the TB germs are cleared from the body. Then the TB germs multiply again. It's therefore important people take medications till they are told they are cured!

2. The giving of lower doses

3.Giving less combinations of drugs to treat TB...Normally, TB patients take up to 4 different drugs, or in combination tablets (not two or three!)

4. Sometimes one can be exposed to a person already suffering from MDR-TB

When is MDR-TB suspected?

1. A person with usual TB does not improve while on treatment, continues to have cough, night sweats and fevers, loss of weight.

2. If TB germs are found in one's sputum even when taking drugs well for two months

3. When 6 months down the treatment lane one is still passing TB germs in sputum

4. When a person caring for a TB patient or stays with a TB patient and starts to cough

note: the lab tests can take up to 3 months to complete, and MDR TB, is deadly if not attended to!

How to prevent MDR-TB

1.Take drugs as instructed by health workers for normal TB

2. Covering one's mouth or use of hand kerchiefs to cover the mouth when in public places/ around people having chronic coughs.

3 People on treatment for TB should keep their windows always open to allow fresh air to circulate
4. The care of suspects and patients in isolated facilities where possible.
5. Family members must sleep in separate rooms when caring for patients of MDR-TB
6. Adopt a healthy life style-eating well, physical exercises, avoid alcohol, smoking.

How long is treatment for MDR-TB?
Treatment can take up to 18-24 months, otherwise if treated less time, it can return.

Can MDR-TB be treatable?
The short answer is YES! But the diagnosis must be taken early and treatment started without delay!

Conclusions
MDR-TB symptoms are the same as for the usual TB. MDR-TB can only be confirmed by lab tests, not symptoms!

79. Anaemia

Anaemia or "little blood" can be understood to mean a reduction in red blood cell mass. We all know that the red cells contain a substance called haemoglobin, the substance that helps the cells carry oxygen to different organs in the body.

Red cells are manufactured in the bone marrow and their grave yard is the spleen. A spleen is a pearl shaped organ in the left flank of the abdomen.
Red cells normally live in the body for 120 days, after which new cells are produced from a combination of bile, iron and globin, a protein. The whole process being controlled by a chemical from the kidneys called Erythropoietin. Erythropoietin is essentially a hormone... A hormone is a chemical produced in minute doses in several organs. Examples of hormones we commonly meet in practice are Oestrogen, progesterone, thyroxin from the thyroid gland, adrenaline from the adrenal gland.

So, anaemia then is any reduction due to any reason of the blood cell mass. Common reason for anaemia is bleeding or loss of white blood cells and reduced production of red blood cells. Blood loss can be as a result of heavy menstruation, growth in the womb or fibroids, womb infections, general sickness of a woman whereas increased destruction of red cells can be a result of infection such as malaria, HIV or some virus causing what is called haemolytic (result of break down); this is usually an iron deficiency anaemia. Chemicals or drugs can also

lead to reduced destruction of red cells, as well.
Reduced production of red blood cells can be a result of cancer of the bone marrow or blood, lack or reduced vitamins intake (folic acid, B12, Iron etc.) or x- ray destruction of the bone marrow. Sometimes anaemia can be due to poor diet as a whole and/or poor absorption of the iron in the stomach, for any other reason like gastritis or other. Kidney disease, can also be a cause for anaemia's rare cause is what I have seen only once in 30 yrs. (and we were all very much baffled to make a diagnosis once!) can be the increased work of the spleen or hyper -splenism, for reasons one cannot explain!

What is important to remember is that anaemia is never a diagnosis, there is always a cause for it. Anaemia alone does not say much about why the condition is present in the body. So, anaemia is not a disease as such but a sign of a disease the person with anaemia easily feels tired, appears pale or white, has heart palpitations, develops shortness of breath or experiences fainting episodes as well as headaches. An anaemic person is more prone to develop different infections in the body.

A simple haemoglobin blood estimation is usually carried out to confirm a diagnosis of anaemia, but a lot more complicated investigation is needed to explain the cause for it.
Treatment, therefore, is aimed at the cause. It is therefore, wrong to think that every anaemic patient needs replacement of iron tablets as is often taken for

granted by most people. Only the anaemia that is iron deficient type would benefit from a supply of exogenous iron. Some may need other components like folic acid, vitamin B 12 preparations or other drugs. In extreme cases, blood is given to correct the problem of anaemia. Special mention here should be made about the relative anaemia in pregnancy. It's very rare to find a haemoglobin in a pregnant woman of above 16(normal values for HB are 14-18, add or remove 1 from both ends). In pregnancy, there is what we call heamo dilution, which is a physiological dilution of the amount of blood in the body due to the increase in fluid levels brought about the pregnancy, this coupled with increased intake of blood components by the growing foetus. However, the approach in this one, is better left to specialist women doctors!

80. Throw away that cough mixture!

The so- called cough remedies deserve special discussion today, have you ever wondered why you never get to be given some in hospitals or clinics, well at least, for the past twenty yrs. or so? Yes, of course, cough remedies are plenty in private chemists, pharmacies and clinics, perhaps even in some private hospitals. The reasons for this is easy to understand! But am not about getting lynched by these fellows dishing out these things, but i truly hope they don't do that to your children! Let them do that to your grownups, because you never ever want to listen to medical sense sometimes! Good luck!

Cough mixtures can broadly be understood to belong to two groups, those that work as expectorants and those that work as suppressants. Expectorants increase the fluidity of bronchial secretions, whereas suppressants are drying agents which prevent secretions altogether or they may work on the cough reflex suppressing such.

With regard to expectorants, it is unfortunate fact that all infants and small children, with bronchitis (cough, dry or wet, without fever) tend to over secrete mucus and can even drown themselves in it. This then becomes clear to any one that were they doing what they are assumed to do, they would bring more problems to the coughing patient, but fortunately, most of them are inert. Some even contain codeine, you wouldn't want near your child or yourself!

Cough suppressants if they worked, would prevent the clearing of the very mucus we don't want, in the throat of a coughing patient, and "drowning" would follow.

So now let me shock you today, by telling you the truth that cough mixtures, all cough mixtures, if they did what they are supposed to, would be lethal! Fortunately, though, they are without effect and you had better know that they are nothing more than placebo medications (A placebo is any medication or substance that is claimed to do what it does not do, and mostly are not dangerous. Most work thru a psychological line!)

So now can you throw away that cough mixture you are keeping in your house, please! So sorry to disappoint you, please forgive me!

81. Teething!

This has been the subject of unnecessary controversy and am afraid nonsense, then any topic I know in medicine!
If you look in the mouth of an infant, between the ages of three months and three years, you will be able to see a tooth that " is just about to come thru, is just coming thru, or has just come thru. 'Please don't attribute a child's problems to this. Teething contrary to your grandmother's advice does not cause pain, insomnia. Indigestion, diarrhoea, vomiting, convulsions, abdominal pains or discomfort, not even fever!
A wise general principle is to assume that teething produces nothing but teeth. Now don't ask me why there are" medications" for teething being sold, you never get this in any hospital!
Of course staining of teeth can be caused by the injudicious administration of Tetracycline (antibiotic) in a child. In fact, such should not be given to a child less than eight year of age! Or sometimes the staining of teeth can be due to a high level of bilirubin, a compound found in red blood cells. Blood cells can break up at an increased rate in such cases as severe malaria or liver disease.
So, no, teething does not cause any problems to a growing child!

82.   Warts

Thanks to ARVT, the incidence of warts is greatly reduced. You may not believe it, but vaginal warts and penile warts had given us a run for our money in the 80'sand early 90's. This is the time when we lost close ones to HIV in doves, this is the time when ARVT was still unavailable or way too expensive for most people to even be put on it.
We have come from very far, from using ineffective anti-cancer drugs, to using mono therapy, dual therapy to the now effective triple therapy. This is why most doctors don't want to tolerate those traditional healers wanting to play therapists for HIV-or even some lawyers! Neither do we tolerate faith healers, prophets as far as the scourge is concerned. But let me not digress! I wanted to talk about warts.
Warts can grow anywhere, mostly found on private parts, the scientific name is *Condylomata acuminate* and are caused by human papilloma virus-HPV (there are many types of such viruses!). The same type that causes cancer of the cervix. Transmitted by contact and thru blood. Most often, it comes under the heading of sexually transmitted infections. Warts like TB, have always been there since time immemorial, but with the advent of HIV which reduces the body immunity, we have seen more and more cases. So it would be a good idea to test for HIV for anyone having warts! Just like we do for Tuberculosis. Warts look like some vegetative growth, may easily bleed when handled roughly, they don't actually pain unless and

until secondary infection does crop in or they spread to surrounding organs. Most of them are slow growths, but in pregnancy have a tendency to really grow very fast. Treatment is by creams like podophyllin, podotoxin, which may dissolve the lesions. But when massive may require surgery - cutting and electrical cauterization. In men, sometimes circumcision is resorted to when they grow on the prepuce.
Warts may often recur!

83. Cigarettes and pregnancy.

Cigarette smoke contains tar, irritants, carbon monoxide and nicotine which are harmful. Of these, carbon monoxide and nicotine enters the mother's blood if she smokes and may cross the placenta into the foetus blood stream. They have a reduction effect on birth weight, the conditions described as intra-uterine growth retardation (IUGR). IUGR can be a cause of premature birth.
Nicotine cause vasoconstriction and therefore reduce blood flow through the placenta. This may affect development of the blood vessels in the umbilical cord and placenta.
Carbon monoxide reduces the oxygen carrying capacity of haemoglobin. This may have effects on the foetus.

84. The truth about injections!

Ati *"mwana ense odwala diarrhoea, now is okay after the Dr. or nurse gave it injection!"* Loosely interpreted as, '*The child had diarrhoea, only became better after it was given injection!"*
Wrong...injections are used only for:

1. Seriously vomiting patients
2. Extremely sick patients unable to take oral drugs
3 in rare cases when doctors want to get the drug to act quickly, because oral takes about 40 minutes for a drug to get absorbed into the blood, whereas injections take seconds, however, the period of action would be the same!

4. Some intra muscular injections are used for their depot effect, i.e. releasing the active ingredients slowly over time and not because they are better! e.g. Depo Provera for contraception.

5 The truth is, oral is always the best, unless not possible, it's less expensive, does not require trained hands, even when there is some vomiting, believe me, something will still remain inside!

6 Diarrhoea is rarely a condition needing injection treatment! Only give the body the required lost fluids, for it to sort itself out! When there is need for drugs, the oral route is always the best!

85. Just so you do not forget!

1. There is no such thing as organ enlargement using some herbs or tablets. The stuff you keep seeing on flyers inviting you to pay for such, is all just crap! Neither is there such things as colon cleansing or detoxifying! Your body has in built mechanisms for such-the lungs, the kidneys, the rectum, your skin!

2. Cough-Not every cough requires any antibiotic like your Amoxillins, Septrins, Erythromycins or Penicillin V. In fact, most coughs are dry and they require no treatment at all, not even cough mixtures. The less you misuse antibiotics the better for every one of us to preserve the activity of the drugs when we really need to use them. In other words, you help prevent resistance to drugs.

3. Chloroquine, Fansidar are no longer used to treat malaria for the same above reasons! The present drug Cuoartem (Arthemether) is expensive, so is quinine for severe and cerebral malaria. We are paying for our own sins!

4. Neither do you or your child having short lived diarrhoea in need of Flagyl, Septrins or other antibiotics. Use simple rehydration with ORS to replace lost fluids and the diarrhoea will stop eventually.

5. Pray if you want to, but don't think some prophet can make you get rich, through miracle money, or treat your diseases ...remember most diseases do indeed heal themselves, that's no miracle! When in doubt go ask the

health worker, just like you take your car to the mechanic when it has a fault! (Not to your prophet!)

6. Do not force your child, sister, brother or any relative choose their career for the sake of your wishes. It's their life, let them choose what is closer to their hearts. It's their life, you won't always be there! And remember there is no such thing as a better profession, just different ones. Success in anything is more to do with passion and loving one's job, than anything else!

7. As a parent, remember to start training your child in whatever they may be inherently good at, you will reap a lot from starting them early! In the same vein do not encourage your children to re -sit subjects they are not good in, identify their strengths and forget the rest! Yes, education is important but only if it's the right one, most millionaires are not Ph D holders!
Even selling tomatoes and chicken can get you to heaven, in spite of your degree or diploma! What matters is passion for whatever you put your mind to!

8. Also remember one very crude lesson that love does not pay bills. Keep your head above water. Do not live to satisfy the whole world! Be ready for disappointments and move on! Do not even consider suicide, leave that to the mad fellows!

86 Blood can tell a tale!

1. If it is darkish blue, you have poor oxygen in take
2 if its cherry red of normal consistency, there is adequate oxygen supply to your body
3. If it's watery, or too dilute, you probably are pregnant or have had too much fluid intake
4. Too thick and difficult to move, you have probably got too many red cells (a problem on itself!) or a cancer of the red cells.
5. Too many white cells (the normal being 4000-6000 per ml of blood-you probably have an infection with germs somewhere, and too much of the white cells, could be leukaemia, a form of cancer
6. Too few white cells, you probably have a viral infection or again some cancer-(leukopenia, aplastic anaemia) or your factory has folded or may be under extreme stress from some medications, herbal or conventional.
7. If your tongue or nail beds are pale white, you may have anaemia

8 if you bleed (or prolonged bleeding time) easily from any site, your clotting factors may be in a mess! Severe platelets (cells which help in clotting issues) depletion can lead to this as well

This is the bare minimum that a simple full blood count can show!

87. Basic understanding of fractures

Loosely can be understood as a break in the continuation of the bone architecture or structure.
Am aware that this problem is often misunderstood and sometimes badly treated. The facts are thus:
Causes of fractures;
1. Accidents of different types, falling or being hit by a vehicle, or thru sports activities.
2. Pathological fractures-often this happens in older people without any undue stress as the bones in such people do tend to lose their strength (de -mineralization). In kids up to Primary school going age the site is often the wrist and above the elbow (supracondylar fractures).
Blood vessels are elastic and often escape damage, nerve branches are often small and regrow slowly if given time.
What to expect:
Any fracture if left alone can actually heal, and does heal! The only problem is it may take much longer time and perhaps leave a deformation as the fragments are not well aligned. We have seen this in animals which accidentally break their bones-the fracture do heal.

The other thing is, all bones have blood supply, so there could be bleeding. We know, for example, that pelvic fractures can bleed up to 2 litres of blood which may be not manifest to the outside if the skin is intact over the bones. This can cause extreme shock and sometimes if not corrected in time can lead to death.

Spinal fractures are particularly dangerous with disruption of function and sensation of the organs lower down the fracture site. For this reason, when you find someone in an accident, the best you can do is to avoid moving them about without medical assistance! This i have seen has led to many complications in accident victims in our country! The blood pressure by some reflex mechanism is always dropping in spinal fractures!

Simple fractures- treatment;

-arm sling on the arm to prevent pain by movement

-pain killers are given

-bleeding is stopped by pressure or temporary tying (not more than 2 hrs!) on the limbs

-Then you can have a plaster of Paris fitted or an operation with "nails" to fix the bones is done in a health facility. This is rarely necessary in kids!

-The arm sling or POP (Pilaster of Paris) is kept for three to six weeks in kids, and a bit longer in adults. Nails inserted in adults can be later be removed after healing or left in the bone.

Remember bones heal on their own, so long the fragments are not too far off, and so there is nothing to panic about!

Rib fractures do not need any particular treatment, other than controlling pain! Whereas fractures of the skull bones and face may also be left untouched if they do not lead to too much bleeding into the head, or are not protruding too much down wards to the brain tissue.

Fractures in the leg can be treated for as long as six months or more, but such people often start to move as soon as pain is controlled. Therefore, be wary of prophets who claim all sorts of things Vis a Vis treating of fractures. These people often operate on your ignorance that fractures do heal, if left alone with time!

Fractures in the feet, toes and hands often don't need any particular manipulation, other than controlling pain. Finger fractures may be treated with only bandages or some simple splinting.

88. Pregnancy tips

1. Always register for ANC (Ante Natal Clinic)

2. Every pregnancy has its own tale, do not think you should have had the problem before, when it occurs in your present one

3. Swelling of feet (oedema) is not an ominous sign if not accompanied by changes in BP and proteins in urine.it does not need any treatment but just assurance. Never use drugs that push out water (diuretics) in treating simple oedema!

4. Hypertension in pregnancy must be aggressively addressed, especially if there are proteins in urine (kidney involvement). Progressive rises in BP and proteins in urine in spite of treatment may call for termination or delivery of the pregnancy, regardless of gestation period!

5, Pregnancy may change your food preferences, but eating soil should be discouraged! Soil may contain eggs for worms and may contain very dangerous germs, sometimes.

6 The dictum "once a Caeser, always a Caeser", is an old women's tale, it's not true!

7. No drug is completely safe in pregnancy, except water! It's a matter of weighing the risk Vis a Vis the benefit

8. Other than iron, folic acid, no supplements are necessary in pregnancy

9. There is always a drop in the haemoglobin levels in any pregnancy, but it should not be too high. The reason is that there is haemo- dilution (blood dilution) with increased fluid in any pregnancy

10. Diabetes in pregnancy, Pregnancy induced hypertension and Isoimmunisation (ABO, blood group incompatibility) should never ever be taken up to term for delivery. Delivery must be effected by 37 weeks gestation by the most appropriate means.

89. Ultra -sound or scanning in pregnancy

Have you ever wondered why some times your request to have a scan in pregnancy at your own time may not be entertained by midwives and doctors? Any investigation is as good as the information it can provide.
A woman would normally have three scans in the nine months barring any problems.
1. Before 12 weeks or three months, a scan is indicated for localization of the pregnancy and determining

gestation period or expected date of delivery. Sometimes used to see if the gestation sac is intact, the number of sacs may be well defined (twins or not)

2. 20 weeks-24 weeks (the period when late abortions can be entertained. Here the organs of the baby are well defined-the spine, the kidneys, the heart. Neuro abnormalities or any other abnormalities can easily be seen. The position of the foetus is immaterial, as it swims in a pool of liquor (water, not alcohol!) and may change position as often as it wants. Expected date of delivery is well defined by the scan. Investigations like amniocentesis, the study of the state of liquor and indirectly foetus are often may be done. Placental location is often irrelevant to continued care, as there is no labour!
Sex determination of the baby is possible but often not an indication to demand a scan (unless of course you are Indian, who culturally we are told may loathe female foetuses).In Zambia , one would think it's an irrelevant issue ,as you can do very little about it, am told you have unisex clothes early in life!

3 After 37-38 weeks to plan mode of delivery as placental position won't change, the size of baby changes little, the position in the womb is fixed. The amount of liquor and condition or activity of the foetus is documented. Size of baby is automatically measured. One thing though size should be relative to maternal pelvis!

90. Tongue tie

I feel like addressing this once again!

Believe me, this condition does not exist, unless iatrogenic ally caused by cutting short the tongue in cases of children with a tendency to keloid formations. The truth is the anterior third of the tongue is just short or missing or is small. With time, the tongue if left alone grows out and the so-called tongue tie retracts. It's surprising how our grandmothers seem to be all knowing in diagnosing problems in the mouth! Fortunately, though, the unnecessary operation of cutting the so-called tie does not leave any permanent damage. However, no treatment is really required except to keep the surgeon well away! i can vouch that the mothers i duly advised to leave their children alone in my practice, never ever complained again, as long as they received proper counselling!

<u>Penicillin revolutionized medicine!</u>
When George Bush went after Saddam Hussein in Iraq many people got injured in battle. Without the use of penicillin during surgeries like amputations and abdominal injuries many could have kicked the bucket!
Penicillin happens to be the first naturally occurring agent that turned the world of infections upside down. Accidentally discovered by a Lab Technician working on the flu virus, Sir Alexander Fleming. This drug has made us treat Gonorrhoea, syphilis, endocarditis (inflammation of the "inside" of the heart), meningitis, pneumonia which previously would kill people in -mass. Fleming discovered

this drug from a mould that grew accidentally on a growth of bacteria in his lab in London.

Now for those getting all excited about how plants can give you medicines, read this...

1. He was a lab technician, not a lawyer, already studying diseases!

2. He was working in a well-equipped lab in London

3. His medicine only knew wide spread use after 1942! He discovered it in 1928!

4. Laboratories had to come in with scientists to work out extraction of the active ingredient, the doses and the like

5. Fleming did not use anecdotes of successes to convince the world!

The Tongue as a window!

I recall one of my professors saying that he could tell you about your health by looking at your tongue. I thought he was a big joke, but having practiced close to three decades, the old fellow was right! Believe what his old brain was hinting as I joined him with white hair!

1. White tongue or pale one-shows you have anaemia or little blood

2. A red tongue may show you have too much blood or red blood cells

3 A yellow coat -would show liver derangement or infection like malaria or inflammation of the liver-hepatitis or even a liver cancer-hepatoma or your gall bladder output may be blocked by a stone or growth in its ducts.

4. A white coat- May suggest a digestive problem

5.A dry tongue may suggest dehydration

6. A geographic tongue, with lines like a map, though people might think is a problem actually does not mean a thing!

Now I know experience is the best teacher! Nothing beats experience!

91. Iatrogenic illness

Most people know, except perhaps prophets, it's a sobering thought that most sick people in fact do recover without any treatment at all. Health workers know this very well, that's why sometimes they give you worthless medications (but harmless ones) knowing very well you will recover. Some people may think and attribute this to miracles but the truth is, the body is always the best doctor!

Sometimes some people think injections heal better than tablets, also not exactly true. Just like the feeling that the bitter the medications, the better it is! This is often used by traditional healers to their advantage!

So Iatrogenic illnesses are the ones healers bring about to you in their search for "better treatments" that may not have a medical basis, or sometimes side effects of doing too much of anything as relates to investigations and treatment strategies that may be undertaken by a health worker. Which cases come to mind?

1. Tonsillectomy (removal of tonsils)-I will surprise you, this operation is often unnecessary. Apart from the tragedy of those who actually die from the operation,

there is no evidence, am afraid, to show that the survivors derive any benefit that might compensate the bereaved!
2. Intravenous fluids or what in Zambia, we call "drips". Drips, you might want to know carry risks. Of course, the benefits of drips far outweigh the dangers but a wrong electrolyte not indicated can cause a lot of damage, all the way to over loading the heart and lungs! Or an infection can be introduced thru the skin to the body!

3 X /ray-Please don't force your way to getting unnecessary x rays, it could be the difference for a future cancerous growth in years to come. Or it could affect your fertility! Let me add that to do an x ray when not indicated is negligent, but also not to do an x/ray when it is indicated is also negligent!

4 Tongue ties- The cutting of the supposed tongue tie in a talking child is a misnomer of treatment, Tongue ties do not really exist, except for the grandmothers!
Let me close by saying that health workers have always to ask themselves whether the treatment or investigations they order on a patient are really necessary or they aren't. This is the only way to avoid iatrogenic illnesses.

92. Multi-Drug Resistant TB (MDR-TB

What is it?
Normally all TB is treatable, but when it is resistant to the two common drugs normally used to treat it-Isoniazid and Rifampicin. TB germs become resistant when they cannot be eradicated effectively in spite of treatment. The symptoms for this type of TB is however the same as the normal TB and can only be confirmed by lab tests.

How does one get it?
1. Stopping treatment before being told to do so-most people with TB feel better two weeks after starting treatment for TB and therefore may feel like stopping the drugs on their own, before in reality all the TB germs are cleared from the body. Then the TB germs multiply again. It's therefore important people take medications till they are told they are cured!
2. The giving of lower doses
3.Giving less combinations of drugs to treat TB. Normally TB patients take up to 4 different drugs, or in combination tablets (not two or three!)
4. Sometimes one can be exposed to a person already suffering from MDR-TB

When is MDR-TB suspected?
1. A person with usual TB does not improve while on treatment, continues to have cough, night sweats and fevers, loss of weight.
2. If TB germs are found in one's sputum even when taking drugs well for two months
3. When 6 months down the treatment lane one is still

passing TB germs in sputum
4. When a person caring for a TB patient or stays with a TB patient and starts to cough
note: The lab tests can take up to 3 months to complete, and MDR TB, is deadly if not attended to!

How to prevent MDR-TB
1.Take drugs as instructed by health workers for normal TB
2. Covering one's mouth or use of hand kerchiefs to cover the mouth when in public places/ around people having chronic coughs.
3 People on treatment for TB should keep their windows always open to allow fresh air to circulate
4. The care of suspects and patients in isolated facilities where possible.
5. Family members must sleep in separate rooms when caring for patients of MDR-TB
6. Adopt a healthy life style-eating well, physical exercises, avoid alcohol, smoking.

How long is treatment for MDR-TB?
Treatment can take up to 18-24 months, otherwise if treated less time, it can return.

Can MDR-TB be treatable?
The short answer is YES! But the diagnosis must be taken early and treatment started without delay!

Conclusions
MDR-TB symptoms are the same as for the usual TB.

MDR-TB can only be confirmed by lab tests, not symptoms!

<u>Why you should never ever contemplate drinking some concoctions in order to procure abortion...</u>
1.When you take water, any fluid or drug, it of course, goes into the stomach, then to the liver to be broken down or stored, then onto the kidneys thru blood... and lungs for expulsion.
2. Now anything passing the liver thru blood has to pass thru your heart, and then to the brain...and this is where the worst can happen! Depending on the strength you are likely to damage your brain cells (encephalopathy)...not to talk of the adverse effects on your liver and kidneys!

3. Then only does your medicine produce a toxicity on the womb thru blood, your womb may lose the contents, but not before you are too sick or almost dead!

4. Other means like introducing pens or other foreign objects have a direct danger of introducing infection or perforating the intestines which lie next to the womb. The infection can have immediate complications like spreading or can work way afterwards blocking your tubes (infertility). The other danger may be serious bleeding from the sudden detachment of harming of the inside walls of the womb!
Medicines can have multiple effects on the body, so it's not safe to take anything which has no selective action on the womb! This is the danger of all the strong teas, and other concoctions we hear about! Keep away!
Note: Medications used in hospitals and procedures for planned abortions take all this in cognizance! The Drs.

know the selective action of the drug being given, and they know the anatomy if instruments are used!

Getting things into perspective!
You may have heard the following medical insights that you should not sleep on your right side of your body because

1. Sleeping on the right may lead to oesophageal reflux as the oesophagus or food pipe enters the stomach from the right top; making acid easier to climb up your throat, makes digestion of food much more difficult, and may cause pain along the throat.

2. The heart works better pumping blood to the rest of the body as the aorta, the largest blood vessel, bends to the left as it leaves the heart.

3. The main body of the stomach lies more on the left side, lying on the right side may push the stomach against the pancreatic duct from the pancreases, which makes it difficult for the flow of the pancreatic juice (for digestion of food) and other medical hacks

But the truth is neither is sleeping mouth up good for a long time as the tongue may fall behind the throat obstructing your breathing. But also sleeping on the left may impede lymph circulation as the main lymph vessels pass on the left. The spleen lies on the left as well, pressure on it may impede its work of blood cell regulation. The lymphatic system is like a cleaner or drainage system in your body.

Don't worry, the body is a clever machine and unless you are comatose or too drunk, change of position happens in the night automatically without you even being aware of it. But remember prolonged use of one side may lead to bed sores and body aches-especially in those who are unconscious. The rule is to change position every two hours at least.

93. Bad habits die hard!

1. It does not matter what we tell you about the benefits of circumcision, the danger of human papilloma virus vis a vis cervical cancer, and that the HPV dwells under the fore skin...people want to continue singing the old songs. Look, we have new data, information has improved on HIV...no, you still think its western vs. African politics!
2. However, many times we preach about the need for lumber puncture for the proper diagnosis and treatment of meningitis, we seem to be hitting a black hole, people still want to believe lumber puncture and not meningitis is the cause of deaths. Once again tell your relatives that meningitis can kill rather very fast, and it may be bacterial, fungal or viral, or even tuberculosis, hence the need for lumber puncture to see which organisms may be responsible, so doctors my aim their weapons against them, the earlier it is done the better for the patient!
So one more time, have you changed your mind? Tell us what you think!
3. ARVT has "saved" lives, improved the life expectancy of many nations yet many out there still think, the African has found a cure for HIV, even though the rest of the whole world is still grappling for a vaccine and cure! Some

still think HIV is a lab engineered virus against the blacks (in spite of the fact that the whole world has been affected by it), yet others still dream HIV and AIDS are not related! The amount of ignorance is just amazing!

94. The Cold Season is here!

Let us recap how to navigate thru it, at least medically speaking!
1. Don't take cough mixtures for every cough, take warm fluids, soothing throat things like warm honey. Let cough run its course, it is there to defend you (it's a defence mechanism employed by your body against irritants)
2.But a cough more than two weeks may need medical attention, to rule out some serious infection, especially if it comes with fever or bloody sputum, or it is a wet cough.
3.A small child need to be kept warm all the time, any refusal of feeds, with or without fever, any lethargy, may indicate serious disease and needs a doctors to see.
4 Avoid buying antibiotics and using them without prescription from a dr. and also suspect malpractice when the same is given to you by any health worker for simple (uncomplicated) flu.
5 Don't get excited by flu jabs...you are unlikely to protect yourself from catching flu, as the flu jabs cannot cover all possible (viral) causes of flu
4.Pneumonia is a serious ailment, especially in children,

and may require admission to a health facility. But not every cough is pneumonia! It could be viral, fungal or bacterial or even chemical as in inhalation of toxic fumes ...fever is always present in most cases of pneumonia.

5 Not every sore throat requires medications, mostly are viral, soothe the throat, avoid cold drinks and wait for nature to sort you out!
6 Above all remember common cold, flu are viral infections, please do not use antibiotics!

95. Clear "donts" in medicine...

1. Do not use other people's medical complaints and fears as exactly the same as yours, as no two people are exactly the same. The stories of "such and such had the same problem", should be taken with a pinch of salt!

2 First line of treatment for any worrying diarrhoea is always fluids/ water. ORS...Not antibiotics. Even in cases where there is vomiting something gets retained! Long standing diarrhoea with mucus or blood needs to be investigated by a dr.

3. Avoid painting the head as traditional treatment in *diarrhoearing* small children whose anterior fontanel (Space in the centre of the head) is sunken and there is pulsating of the top of the head. This traditional approach is dangerous, as it wastes time, and the child may lose more fluids and become weaker!

4. Likewise discourage sitting small children with diarrhoea in concoctions as treatment. The anus is pretty fast in absorbing toxic medicines and your child may become worse!

5 Don't take tablets you are told to be taken on a full stomach on an empty tummy, you may induce nausea and vomiting. Also, don't take tablets you are told are to be taken on an empty stomach (usually two hrs. after eating) on a full tummy, you may slow their action

7. Patients with gastritis/stomach ulcers, bleeding tendencies should avoid aspirin, so are those with bronchial asthma

8. Remember the safest drug in pregnancy is water! Always consult your health worker for advice!

9. Never ever fear blood transfusions for yourself, your relative or child, it can save one's life. Don't mix religious beliefs with life saving measures!

10 Medicine is never learnt from Google, leave controversial topics like masturbation, circumcision, family planning, infertility issues, sexual problems to the experts, they are better informed to guide you sieve sense from nonsense. Don't assume all you read to be true on Google!

96. Infertility issues

I have noticed many questions related to this, even though we had discussed it on this forum before. Looks like we have many customers out there. So here is some food for you today!

First and foremost bareness or infertility can only be talked about if the following are in place...

1.One year of trying to conceive

2. Regular exposure to sex

 Pregnancy does not follow every exposure to sex. A woman releases eggs only once a month, so called fertile period does not necessarily result in one getting pregnant, as other issues may be at play.

What is regular sex-At least 2-3 days in week is presumed normal. Am not talking of rounds here but days! Too regular intercourse is not also advisable as the quantity of semen in the man may not be optimal. A man needs days to make up the required quantity, more so if age is advanced!

Causes of infertility-related to woman is about 50%, man 40% and a combination of both at 10 %. So the habit of blaming the woman as the cause for infertility practiced in most of our homes is not sensible! In fact, this can be secondary as when one had child before and primary as when no child was conceived before. In Zambia though, most cases of infertility are related to blocked fallopian tubes in the woman, followed by hormonal changes, obesity, and secondary to a chronic disease like TB, do not forget the role of stress in regulating the menses in the woman!

Man-normal quantity of semen is around a ml or two, 50-250 000 000 sperms or so in one ml, and the sperms should not have abnormalities like double heads, should swim normally. In most cases that's all a man needs to have checked. The dr. will then check for possible causes if sperms are reduced in quantity or absent (I won't go into details here)

The woman on the other hand should have the following checked...

1. A full blood count- to look for anaemia
2. An examination for syphilis (RPR) and other STDs
3. A urine test - to check for any infections
4.A scan- to check for the size of ovaries and any possible cysts
5 A hormone profile
6.An HSG-Hystero- Salpingography- Special x-ray to check for the permeability of tubes
7 Additional investigations according to clinical findings like skull x-rays, thyroid function, ovulation tests etc.

Treatment is aimed at the cause, and can vary from...

-Assurance to control stress issues
-Treating infections and correcting weight problems as well as anaemia
-counselling and acceptance of the situation
-Hormonal provision
-Adoption
-Tubal surgery in woman(very poor success rate), urological surgery in man
-Artificial insemination-a bit expensive, done in RSA)

97. Fibroid Uterus (womb), revisited.

Muscular growth from the womb or on the womb muscles. Causes not well understood, but sometimes hormonal changes may be implicated.
Fibroids are not cancerous, but rarely may turn to cancer (please rarely!)
types- depends on where they are found...
-Cervical
-Sub mucosal-within the womb space
-Sub-serous-on top of the outside muscle of the womb
-intramural-within the musculature of the womb
Therefore symptoms or complaints will depend on location. Won't discuss cervical, as they are very rare
1. When they grow within the space inside-prolonged heavy periods, abortions, periods with heavy clots. Fertility may be affected
2. When they grow on top- periods not affected, may give pain when the press on surrounding organs like bladder and colon, nerves. Some complaints are related to just how big they become, urinary dribbling when they press on bladder for example. Pain when they grow towards nerves in abdomen. Fertility not affected.
3 In the muscle-heavy periods, prolonged periods, Pain when the womb grows too much. Fertility may be affected thru abortions, or disorganizing the function of the fallopian tubes by kinking them or blockage,
diagnosis- by vaginal examination and ultra sound-rays are useless!

Note: when the woman is approaching menopause, may reduce in size!

Treatment-is mostly removal of fibroids by cutting them off or inoculation or myomectomy where possible or total removal of the womb when the whole womb is affected (hysterectomy)
Please note- fibroids cannot be treated by prophets!!Sorry to say i have had patients going to Nigeria for this! Its unwise and a waste of time!

98. Bizarre gynae disease

It's of course Endometriosis!
First, understand that the womb as being made out of three layers. Well not exactly, but almost. The inner is called endometrium, the one which sheds during menses, the outer is the myometrium, and the surrounding cellulose tissue the parametrium which "houses" the ovary and tubes. So the word endometriosis comes from the inner aspect of the womb-endometrium!
Imagine during periods you get all sorts of pains in different sites in the body. This could be that the body at birth had run away endometrial tissues depositing themselves all over. When the main body bleeds, so do the "kids! 'It is this bleeding that causes pains from irritations in different sites in your body! Fallopian tubes may get disorganized leading to infertility. This is the strange condition we call endometriosis, a very difficult condition to diagnose and treat.

Diagnosis is by history and laparoscopic investigations
(and how many centres, have this laparoscopy, let alone
the necessary training of staff),
In the years gone by, we used to use the drug Danazol, for
treatment of endometriosis but then newer drugs are
being introduced, and it would not be in your interest or
mine to go further than this!

99. Is urine safe to treat your wounds?

Legend has it that urine has been used before to treat
wounds. Stranded soldiers have been known to buy time
by drinking own urine. Some naturalists advise drinking
own urine to cure cancer!
Of course if the only fluid available is urine, we can't argue
with you, you got to survive. Just like stranded sea men
are told not to drink sea water (because of salts) but when
the only water which is available is sea water, you would
rather die drinking it!
Urine like faeces is not sterile. Urine is a by-product from
the body, and the body never makes mistakes! If you
think it's cool, try not passing urine for three days! You
will surely die!
So urine on wounds is a risky affair!!

100. Young children do explore!

All kids after two yrs. want to know about their surroundings. The only problem is they do so by taking into the mouth whatever they touch, hence you may get a lot of diarrhoea cases and accidental swallowing of all sorts of objects, in this age group!

Coins, buttons, stones, may be swallowed! Things may be inserted into the ears. Let us talk about the swallowing...

1.Any swallowed object has to pass thru natural constrictions (narrowing) of the gullet or food pipe (or would you rather call it, oesophagus?), first by the entrance to the throat, next where the wind pipe breaks into two (about the middle of your chest), and lastly where the food pipe enters your stomach. Then the object stays there about 4 hrs. And through another constriction enters the colon, if its water or any drink it stays about 40 minutes in the stomach.

2 If the object gets stuck anywhere above the stomach, you will see the child complaining of pain, passing mucus or coughing without end. If it's stuck just by the start of the throat, the object may obstruct the breathing, this becomes a real emergency, and the child may die due to lack of oxygen!

3 What to do?

A-If no signs as above-nothing! The object is likely to come out with stool, at a later time, feed the child normally.

b- If child has difficulty in breathing-turn the child upside down and press hard on its tummy, the object may get dislodged down and out! There may not be enough time to go to or reach a health facility. Or else the object may move allowing the child to breathe a bit (then you have time to run to a health facility!)

c- If child takes passes a lot of mucus from the mouth, develops pain and is crying, but can breathe properly-You have time to take to the health facility

I won't go in details what the health facility will do, instruments exist for extraction, or the child may be referred to a facility able to do this

101. Paraffin ingestion can be fatal!

1. it's colourless like water, and is stored mostly in bottles for the usual drinks. Children may accidentally drink it!
2. It is got dangerous fumes that may enter the respiratory or breathing organs (the bronchus, the lungs). May cause what is called as chemical pneumonia, a very difficult condition to treat, as antibiotics are almost useless!
3. It may be corrosive on the stomach, and food pipe, producing an inflammation or swelling
4. Paraffin can affect the brain by passing thru blood from the stomach, produces collapse and may be even death. There is no dr. or health worker who has not met a child so afflicted, in their practice!

First aid-Don't force vomiting! Give milk and wait if the child is not very sick. If weak, confused, coughing, developing fever rush to a health facility!

A drip at heath facility may help keep the collapse under check, while the body is fighting the intoxication. No attempts are made at stomach wash out-it could be dangerous, as paraffin may affect the respiratory system during the procedure. Treatment is expectant and supportive!
Please do not store paraffin where the child may reach it!

102. Simple guidelines -Men's health

p1. Masturbation- Masturbate if so wish, there is no health risk
2.Men above 40 should have a PSA (Prostate cancer test). It's a quick test but useful
3. Small eruptions around the head-Mostly harmless, sebaceous gland related, if painful and tearing could be herpes genitalis, a self-limiting small infection, will heal with or without acyclovir. Avoid sex during this period, they could be painful and may delay healing!
4 Warts Penile-Go for removal with cream or cautery depending on size, may recur. The cause is human Papilloma Virus (the same one causing cancer in women), Circumcision may be helpful!
Itching/pain on passing urine-may be urinary tract infection, a simple antibiotic may see you thru, but if discharge treat as STD!
6 Painless red sore-Could be a STD, mostly chancre of Syphilis or Chanchroid (cancroid)-go to the clinic!

7 Poor erection / reduced libido-check your age! Stress and tiredness are a major cause. Check your drugs, sugar. Avoid taking Viagra without doctors' prescription, it can be fatal sometimes! Likewise avoid herbs from the street, they never do work! An improvement is often psychological, not herbal related, and you really do not know what else the herb can do in your body!

8. Sex life- Remember, fore play! Think about your partner and not yourself, don't rush and don't stress. If tired or after a quarrel with your partner, don't even try! If things back fire, there is always going to be another day!

103. Simple Guidelines-Women health

1. Discharge vaginal-not every discharge is abnormal, light colourless is a normal finding, which may increase when sexually excited. Candida is may sometimes be in vagina, in very small amounts and should not normally give you any problems, increase in pregnancy or when taking oral combined pills. Should worry you if itching or purulent, frothy. However simple vaginal pessaries can see you through. Discharge of any other colour with any complaints or without should warrant a visit to a health facility.

2, Spotting-this is very mild bleeding from the cervix, vaginal. Hormones (pills) oral ones or injectable ones can give you this. Post-delivery spotting should stop by six weeks. Spotting after cleaning with fingers or sex should (contact bleeding) should warrant a visit for Pap smear or an examination by a health worker.

3 Heavy Periods-Suspect growths in the womb, or a hormonal disturbance

4 Absence of periods (after normal periods)-Suspect stress, injectable contraceptive, pregnancy (sounds foolish, but some women forget!)

5 Lower abdominal pains, with absence of periods-may be an ectopic or pregnancy outside the womb. When no periods missed, think of pelvic inflammatory disease, and rarely sometimes urinary tract infection. Note: STD rarely pains unless it gets complicated!

6 Breast fullness and tenderness-Could be related to an impeding period. Pregnancy does not make painful breasts though they can feel full! Contraceptive pills can be a possibility as well.

7 Small breast mass-if child bearing needs to be assessed by a health worker, especially if painful, Younger ladies below twenty need not worry, could mostly be hormonal! Always make sure your breasts have no sore, are equal, and skin is not indurating in one area

8 Painful Periods-Have no cure! Ignore if not severe or take aspirin to help you cope during periods or just before or shortly after. Panadol is always useless in this!

9 Ultra sound or scanning worries-Most scanners are not gynaecologists and may worry you to death with insignificant diagnosis of cysts. Most women have small cysts, don't you worry to death! Go for follow up! And remember not to read your own scan notes, leave it to the dr., there is a lot the radiographer could misinterpret!

10 Have a pap smear at least two to three yearly if child bearing. It's fast and painless!

104. Nuisance illness!

You wake up to find your private parts painful, all with small red and white dots, some discharging fluid. What to do?
Stop any sexual activity till they heal, wear loose pants or no pants at all! Take pain killers, if you feel like, but not a must. Do not take any antibiotics, they are of no use. Your diagnosis is herpes genitalis, a sort of nuisance but harmless! May take up to a week or more days to heal. Caused by a viral infection, a self-limiting one! Some doctors may advise Acyclovir, some anti-viral drug, but is no cure, may shorten disease progress, just, must be taken very early when the eruptions happen.

105. Alcohol, the facts

Head-It's indeed a stimulant in mild doses but in higher doses is a suppressant. Alcohol is poisonous to brain cells that do not regenerate when they are killed. You have about 100 000 000 000 000 brain cells all in all, maybe that's why you sometimes don't see the damage. Alcohol is a drug, it's addictive; meaning it creates strong craving with repeated over use, and more and higher doses are demanded by the body as use rises. Users become more and more careless to self and responsibilities to care for family drops. Higher doses may result in complete shutdown of the brain activity leading to death.

Chest-The heart muscles suffers, as the heart may become dilated creating a cardiomyopathy, which is another way of saying the heart's contractual powers are decreased as it dilates. Consequently, if the heart cannot pump blood effectively, then the lungs in turn become congested, oedematous or swollen with fluids, you drown in your own fluids! Oxygen supply suffers to the rest of the body and every organ suffers!

Abdomen-The stomach gets hit first producing vomiting as it fights back, eventually it may become inflamed producing gastritis, all the way up to over production of hydrochloric acid and other juices which may eventually cause ulcers or stomach cancer. Then your liver suffers. The liver cells start dying in -mass, as they get poisoned producing inflammation or hepatitis, all the way up to total shrinkage; we call cirrhosis, a condition that is not reversible. Sometimes cancer may develop, Hepatoma as it is called. The early signs of damage to liver cells may be that you develop yellow eyes or jaundice, which itself is a toxin on its own right. The ability of the liver to detoxify your blood plummets flooding the body with unrequited toxic waste. The pancreas a small organ near your stomach that regulates your body sugars through production of insulin and helps in digestion by producing pancreatic juice, may inflame, producing pancreatitis or may become cancerous. Your tummy becomes painful and bigger!

Blood- Your body's production of blood cells suffers as ingredients from the liver/kidneys for the production of blood cells such as erythropoietin and vitamins get depleted. You may develop anaemia or low levels of blood.

Blood vessels- dilate or become bigger under the influence of the toxic effects of alcohol. Your blood pressure drops, oxygen transport to various organs suffers, your organs suffer!

Nerves- Your nerves become more and more paralyzed, penile erections may drop. Frigidity in women may develop. Alcohol as Shakespeare once wrote creates desire but takes away the performance! It is not true that alcohol actually improves sexual performance! Dead nerves don't perform well! Even appetite for food eventually wanes. Driving reactions gets impaired, judgment is messed up, encourages speeding as it gives wrong courage. Common inhibitions break down; our behaviours may become unusual and uncoordinated.

Pregnancy-Alcohol may induce abortions, premature deliveries, may result in brain affected babies at birth. Increased alcohol consumption is a major public health issue of our times. Why then is there so much alcohol in the shops, you might rightly ask?

106. Weight problems revisited!

Weight problems revisited!
Being overweight is a coronary (heart disease) risk, a very high one! The quickest way I would say to reduce your life expectancy is by being obese (and by smoking cigarettes!) This is true for Africa and the world at large, as it is true for our country Zambia.
There are few health conditions that may send us early to meet our maker but are very easy to control. Some conditions just pop out of nothing, and kills us, but weight pops out of our mouths! Many of us though would rather blame the genetics and nature or glands for our being overweight! The truth is the only gland we should be blaming for our being overweight should be our salivary glands! We, the overweight doesn't want to face the truth, we like food too much!
Last time I did research on weight, I found out 95% of obese people have to do with life style problems and only 5% problems can be blamed on genetics and other, causes beyond the control of people. But even this 5% can finally be traced to food intake!
You may recall, we mentioned this early about what obesity is. The best measure is what we call the BMI or Body Mass Index.
BMI= Weight in kg divide by height squared, in metres. So you would end up with values 20-25 as normal
25-30 as overweight
30-35 obese

35-40 grossly obese
Above 40-Morbidly obese (remember morbidity just means sickness!)
You have probably seen adverts for weight reduction which promises results like arithmetic! I mean, if all it took was for you to use some bands and drink yellow or green tea or just drink lemon juice, in order to control your weight, many of these quarks would have been out of business a long time ago! Let me tell you something, weight control is just a matter of diet and exercise, there is no magic wand or tablet or liquid that is going to sort your weight issues permanently!
I should add here also that unless you admit that your mouth and inactivity is to blame, you are not going to solve the weight problem. Don't blame your genes, blame yourself and be ready to change things. I Say so, because in medicine, we know that identical twins separated at birth, which obviously should still have same genes, often have been found to acquire the eating habits of their foster parents, and together with this, develop different weights!
Now, you see, you have some form of thermostat, let us call this your appestat. This is the hypothalamic centre in your brain responsible for your appetite. Its function depends on information learnt over time, information from the nerve endings in your mouth and stomach, the levels of blood sugar in your body. This means that depending on the stimulus or lack of it, the appestat switches off or runs into overdrive! But you see, this control mechanism is automatic, and may misbehave or break down due to inactivity and incorrect eating habits!

I have said it before you have a major problem on your hands if the only muscles you move adequately are only the chewing muscles (the Masseter muscles, as the good dr. will call them)!
So here is what you need to do to control your weight...
1.Take a balanced diet rich in veggies and fruits
2. Don't skip meals-if you skip meals, your body will try to compensate on your next sitting!
3. Exercise regularly-walk. Run, do exercises...anything so long you are active
4. Avoid too much junk fatty foods
5. Avoid overeating

107. Christian Barnard was simply crazy!

Well crazy like Albert Einstein! In a very good way!
He had attended Surgery in USA, learnt his art there and despite the Americans putting in huge sums of money into Cardiac research, he beat them to it, and not only the Americans but the whole World, including the pioneering Russian Heart Surgeons he had visited in 1961, to learn how far they had gone. He did the first successful human heart transplant in the World in 1967! And where? In Africa!
This Cape Town genius did his Masters and Doctorates in Surgery in USA, in just two years, a record few can surpass even today! He then came back to Africa to pioneer some very crazy Surgery that even involved transplanting a head

of a dog to a dog with another head such that the dog had two working heads! His work in Children's surgical diseases was out of this world, as well!

But as most Scientists, (except yours and mine, i hope!) his married life stunk, he married thrice and divorced thrice! He also took too much to the bottle, one wonders if fame had gotten the better of him!

But whatever the case, Barnard's work, has made us appreciate what death really means, that you can have your heart and lungs working but be practically dead-brain dead! Remember the heart he transplanted came from someone you would say then was "alive", his organs were intact, while his brain was dead, following a terrible road accident!

You got to be crazy to put a knife on a pumping heart and "kill" the donor so to say! That was how crazy Christian Barnard was, we shall forever respect him!

Jackie Simukoko: Let me add by saying that the recipient was Louis Washkansky, a 53-year-old grocer with a debilitating
heart condition. Washkansky
received the heart of Denise Darvall, a young woman who was run over by a car on 2
December and had been declared brain dead after suffering serious brain damage. Her father, Edward Darvall agreed to the donation
of his daughter's heart and kidneys. The operation started shortly after midnight on a Saturday night and was completed the next morning
just before 6 a.m. when the new heart in the chest of Louis

Washkansky was electrically
shocked into action. After
regaining consciousness he
was able to talk and on occasion, to walk but his
condition deteriorated and
died of pneumonia eighteen
days after the heart
transplant.

108. Sexual health for men, revisited

Among the more often met problems are 1. Reduced
libido
2.Premature ejaculation
3. Erectile dysfunction. I wish to discuss with you today
Erectile Dysfunction, a problem which affects more than
30% of men between the ages of 40-70 yrs. a problem
that can lead to depression, anxiety, marital discord and
even violence.
Remember that Erectile Dysfunction(ED) is not the same
as reduced libido or premature ejaculation. This is failure
of the man to have adequate erection or the absence of it
to carry out sexual act. In other words,
Most men don't want to talk about it, they regard it as
taboo, or they assume it is normal with advancing age, or
they assume it is all in the mind and never physical. While
some think there is no help that can be given.
Understand erection as simply collection of arterial blood

in the organ that gets trapped for some time, resulting in its rigidity. One can get an erection from
-erotic thoughts
-from genital stimulation
-nocturnal variations/morning erections)
This means that erections can be subjective(by simply thinking) or objective(by stimulation).This then means that ED can be1-Psychological-Where by you want but has no erection or the erection is poor
2-Organic-due to either damaged nerves, damaged blood vessels or damaged penile shaft
How do you tell which is the most likely problem organic or physical or psychological?
The Psychologically induced ED will often mean you don't want but the penis is functional, you are not sexually rousable. Here the night / morning erections will be present. Any of these below can cause psychological ED:
-stress
-depression
-marital disharmony
-feelings of guilty
-feelings of shame
-performance related anxiety
The physical causes can be:
drugs like Digoxin, Beta blockers(like Atropine), Diuretics, Aldomet for BP. Antacids, some pain -killers, obesity ,too much alcohol use and smoking, diseases like hypertension , diabetes, Atherosclerosis, heart failure, etc.
Treatment-if psychogenic may benefit from counselling with or without partner
-Often drugs such as Viagra, Cialis, Levitra are increasingly

used, Intra penile injections, Intra urethral injections, vacuum pumps and prostheses.

All the drugs are take

However, I must warn you drugs such as Viagra are not aphrodiasics, meaning they do not alone make you want sex, you must be aroused first for them to work! This arousal is often by direct stimulation.

Side effects- Headaches, nasal congestion, skin irritations, back pains. Those taking nitrites for heart disease should avoid them. But they work miracles by promoting the production of Nitrous oxide in the penis, a compound responsible for erections.

Drugs should be prescribed by a Dr., and are taken once daily from 30 minutes to 4 hrs. to 12 hrs. before the envisaged sexual act.

About the Author

Doctor Teddy Andrew Mulenga was born in 1958 in the Northern town of Kasama, Zambia. He completed Secondary school at the elite Hillcrest National Technical School in 1978, in Livingstone. After compulsory military training entered the University of Zambia where he majored in Philosophy and Psychology up to 1982 when he won a scholarship to study medicine in the then Soviet Union. He graduated with distinctions in Surgery, Internal medicine, Paediatrics and Obstetrics and Gynaecology. Dr. Mulenga obtained numerous literally certificates during his University studies. His working career took him from Ndola Central hospital to Botswana where he worked for more than 20 years. The author has widely travelled in Europe and Africa which culminated into a high curiosity for human thought and the guest for self- actualization. Dr Mulenga, an avid chess player speaks five languages fluently; English, Russian, Setswana, Bemba and Nyanja. He is now domiciled in the tourist capital of Zambia, Livingstone, and ten minutes' drive from the mighty Victoria Falls. "The Sceptic – "The ABC of Your Health" is his 11th published literally work.

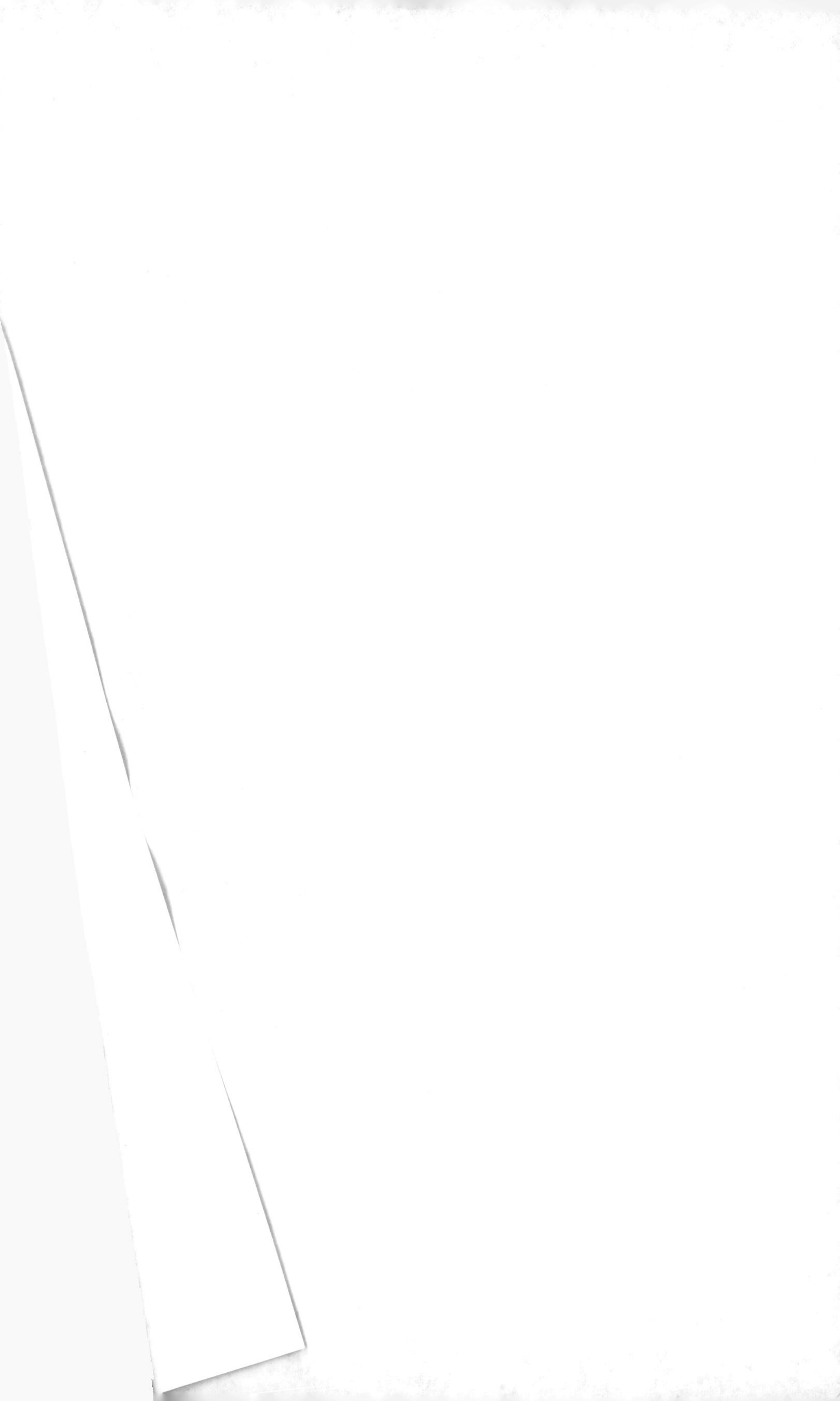